Non-invasive Mechanical Ventilation in Critical Care, Anesthesiology and Palliative Care

Giuseppe Servillo · Maria Vargas
Editors

Non-invasive Mechanical Ventilation in Critical Care, Anesthesiology and Palliative Care

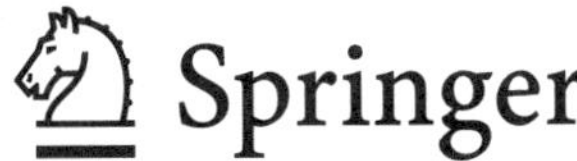

Editors
Giuseppe Servillo
Neurosc, Reprod, Odontostomatol Sc
University of Naples "Federico II"
Naples, Italy

Maria Vargas
Neurosc, Reprod, Odontostomatol Sc
University of Naples "Federico II"
Naples, Italy

ISBN 978-3-031-36512-6   ISBN 978-3-031-36510-2   (eBook)
https://doi.org/10.1007/978-3-031-36510-2

This Springer imprint is published by the registered company Springer Nature Switzerland AG
The registered company address is: Gewerbestrasse 11, 6330 Cham, Switzerland

Contents

Part II   Methodology

5   Why and When to Start Non-invasive Ventilation 37
Greta Zunino, Denise Battaglini, Patricia R. M. Rocco,
and Paolo Pelosi

List of Contributors

Servillo Andrea Department of Ophthalmology, University Vita-Salute, IRCCS Ospedale San Raffaele, Milan, Italy

Anna Annunziata Unit of Respiratory Physiopathology, Monaldi Hospital, Naples, Italy

Stefano Badolato Medicine Ward and Emergency Department, San Giuliano Hospital, Giugliano, Italy

Denise Battaglini Anesthesia and Intensive Care, San Martino Policlinico Hospital, IRCCS for Oncology and Neuroscience, Genoa, Italy
Department of Medicine, University of Barcelona, Barcelona, Spain

Elena Giovanna Bignami Anesthesiology, Critical Care and Pain Medicine Division, Department of Medicine and Surgery, University of Parma, Parma, Italy

C. Brusasco Department of Surgical, Medical, Molecular Pathology and Critical Care Medicine, University of Pisa, Pisa, Italy

Pasquale Buonanno Department of Neurosciences and Reproductive and Odontostomatological Sciences, University of Naples "Federico II", Naples, Italy

Ivana Capuano Department of Neurosciences and Reproductive and Odontostomatological Sciences, University of Naples "Federico II", Naples, Italy

A. Cardu Department of Surgical, Medical, Molecular Pathology and Critical Care Medicine, University of Pisa, Pisa, Italy

Simone Carelli Dipartimento di Scienze dell' Emergenza, Anestesiologiche e della Rianimazione, Fondazione Policlinico Universitario A. Gemelli IRCCS, Rome, Italy

G. Castellano Department of Anesthesia and Intensive Care, Gemelli Molise Hospital, Campobasso, Italy

F. Corradi Department of Surgical, Medical, Molecular Pathology and Critical Care Medicine, University of Pisa, Pisa, Italy

Antonio Coviello Department of Neurosciences, Reproductive and Odontostomatological Sciences, University of Naples "Federico II", Naples, Italy

Salvatore Lucio Cutuli Dipartimento di Scienze dell' Emergenza, Anestesiologiche e della Rianimazione, Fondazione Policlinico Universitario A. Gemelli IRCCS, Rome, Italy

Gennaro De Pascale Dipartimento di Scienze dell' Emergenza, Anestesiologiche e della Rianimazione, Fondazione Policlinico Universitario A. Gemelli IRCCS, Rome, Italy

Facoltà di medicina e chirurgia "A. Gemelli", Università Cattolica del Sacro Cuore, Rome, Italy

Andrea Uriel de Siena Department of Neurosciences and Reproductive and Odontostomatological Sciences, University of Naples "Federico II", Naples, Italy

Maurizio Ferrara Anesthesia and Critical Care, ASL Napoli 1 centro, San Paolo Hospital, Naples, Italy

Giuseppe Fiorentino Unit of Respiratory Physiopathology, Monaldi Hospital, Naples, Italy

F. Forfori Department of Surgical, Medical, Molecular Pathology and Critical Care Medicine, University of Pisa, Pisa, Italy

G. Giuliano Department of Surgical, Medical, Molecular Pathology and Critical Care Medicine, University of Pisa, Pisa, Italy

Ludovica Golino Anesthesia and Intensive Unit of Emergency Department, San Giovanni di Dio Hospital, Frattamaggiore, Italy

Domenico Luca Grieco Dipartimento di Scienze dell' Emergenza, Anestesiologiche e della Rianimazione, Fondazione Policlinico Universitario A. Gemelli IRCCS, Rome, Italy

Carmine Iacovazzo Department of Neuroscience and Reproductive and Odontostomatological Sciences, University of Naples Federico II, Naples, Italy

Department of Neuroscience and Reproductive and Odontostomatological Sciences, Intensive Care Unit, University of Naples Federico II, Naples, Italy

A. Isirdi Department of Surgical, Medical, Molecular Pathology and Critical Care Medicine, University of Pisa, Pisa, Italy

Akarawut Kasemchaiyanun Division of Critical Care Medicine, Department of Medicine Ramathibodi Hospital, Faculty of Medicine Ramathibodi Hospital, Mahidol University, Bangkok, Thailand

Maurizia Lanza Unit of Respiratory Physiopathology, Monaldi Hospital, Naples, Italy

Department of Critical Care, Respiratory Physiopathology, AO dei Colli, Monaldi Hospital, Naples, Italy

Vargas Maria Department of Neurosciences, Reproductive and Odontostomatological Sciences, University of Naples "Federico II", Naples, Italy

A. Marra Department of Neurosciences, Reproductive and Odontostomatological Sciences, University of Naples "Federico II", Naples, Italy

Unit of Anesthesia and Intensive Care, Department of Neurosciences, Reproductive and Odontostomatological Sciences, University of Naples "Federico II", Naples, Italy

Critical Illness, Brain Dysfunction, and Survivorship (CIBS) Center, Vanderbilt University School of Medicine, Nashville, TN, USA

M. Melchionna Clinical Pharmacy Gemelli Molise Hospital, Campobasso, Italy

Raffaele Merola Department of Neurosciences and Reproductive and Odontostomatological Sciences, University of Naples "Federico II", Naples, Italy

V. Motroni Department of Surgical, Medical, Molecular Pathology and Critical Care Medicine, University of Pisa, Pisa, Italy

Serena Nappi Department of Neurosciences and Reproductive and Odontostomatological Sciences, University of Naples "Federico II", Naples, Italy

Angela Pagano Medicine Ward and Emergency Department, San Giuliano Hospital, Giugliano, Italy

L. Palumbo Department of Anesthesia and Intensive Care, Gemelli Molise Hospital, Campobasso, Italy

P. P. Pandharipande Critical Illness, Brain Dysfunction, and Survivorship (CIBS) Center, Vanderbilt University School of Medicine, Nashville, TN, USA

Department of Anesthesiology, Division of Critical Care Medicine, Vanderbilt University School of Medicine, Nashville, TN, USA

Paolo Pelosi Anesthesia and Intensive Care, San Martino Policlinico Hospital, IRCCS for Oncology and Neuroscience, Genoa, Italy

Department of Surgical Sciences and Integrated Diagnostics, University of Genoa, Genoa, Italy

Romina Peroné Anesthesiology Department, Pineta Grande Hospital, Castelvolturno, Italy

Gabriele Pintaudi Dipartimento di Scienze dell' Emergenza, Anestesiologiche e della Rianimazione, Fondazione Policlinico Universitario A. Gemelli IRCCS, Rome, Italy

Erminia Ramponi Medicine Ward and Emergency Department, San Giuliano Hospital, Giugliano, Italy

Marco Rispoli Department of Critical Care, Anesthesia and Intensive Care, AO dei Colli, Monaldi Hospital, Naples, Italy

Patricia R. M. Rocco Laboratory of Pulmonary Investigation, Carlos Chagas Filho Biophysics Institute, Federal University of Rio de Janeiro, Rio de Janeiro, Brazil

Rosario Sara Department of Neuroscience and Reproductive and Odontostomatological Sciences, University of Naples Federico II, Naples, Italy

Andrea Servillo Department of Ophthalmology, University Vita-Salute, IRCCS Ospedale San Raffaele, Milan, Italy

Giuseppe Servillo Department of Neuroscience and Reproductive and Odontostomatological Sciences, University of Naples Federico II, Naples, Italy
Department of Neuroscience and Reproductive and Odontostomatological Sciences, Intensive Care Unit, University of Naples Federico II, Naples, Italy

Ezio Spasari Anesthesia and Intensive Unit of Emergency Department, San Giovanni di Dio Hospital, Frattamaggiore, Italy

Francesco Squillacioti Department of Neurosciences and Reproductive and Odontostomatological Sciences, University of Naples "Federico II", Naples, Italy

Yuda Sutherasan Division of Pulmonary and Pulmonary Critical Care Medicine, Department of Medicine Ramathibodi Hospital, Faculty of Medicine Ramathibodi Hospital, Mahidol University, Bangkok, Thailand

E. Taddei Department of Surgical, Medical, Molecular Pathology and Critical Care Medicine, University of Pisa, Pisa, Italy

Eloisa Sofia Tanzarella Dipartimento di Scienze dell' Emergenza, Anestesiologiche e della Rianimazione, Fondazione Policlinico Universitario A. Gemelli IRCCS, Rome, Italy

Pongdhep Theerawit Division of Critical Care Medicine, Department of Medicine Ramathibodi Hospital, Faculty of Medicine Ramathibodi Hospital, Mahidol University, Bangkok, Thailand

Loredana Tibullo Medicine Department, San Giuseppe Moscati Hospital, Avellino, Italy

D. Vannini Department of Surgical, Medical, Molecular Pathology and Critical Care Medicine, University of Pisa, Pisa, Italy

Joel Vargas Dipartimento di Scienze dell' Emergenza, Anestesiologiche e della Rianimazione, Fondazione Policlinico Universitario A. Gemelli IRCCS, Rome, Italy

Maria Vargas Department of Neurosciences, Reproductive and Odontostomatological Sciences, University of Naples "Federico II", Naples, Italy

Department of Neuroscience and Reproductive and Odontostomatological Sciences, Intensive Care Unit, University of Naples Federico II, Naples, Italy

Nicola Vargas Medicine Ward and Emergency Department, San Giuliano Hospital, Giugliano, Italy

Claudia Veropalumbo Department of Neuroscience and Reproductive and Odontostomatological Sciences, University of Naples Federico II, Naples, Italy

Department of Neuroscience and Reproductive and Odontostomatological Sciences, Intensive Care Unit, University of Naples Federico II, Naples, Italy

Greta Zunino Anesthesia and Intensive Care, San Martino Policlinico Hospital, IRCCS for Oncology and Neuroscience, Genoa, Italy

Department of Surgical Sciences and Integrated Diagnostics, University of Genoa, Genoa, Italy

Abbreviations

A/C	Assist/Control
ACPE	Acute cardiogenic pulmonary edema
ARDS	Acute respiratory distress syndrome
ARF	Acute respiratory failure
ASA	American Society of Anesthesiologists
BiPAP	Bi-level positive airway pressure
BNP	B-type natriuretic peptide
COPD	Chronic obstructive pulmonary disease
CPAP	Continuous positive airway pressure
CT	Computed tomography
EAdi	Electrical activity of the diaphragm
ED	Emitted dose
ED	Emergency department
EPAP	Expiratory positive airway pressure
ETI	Endotracheal intubation
EVLW	Extravascular lung water
FEV1	Forced expiratory volume in 1 s
FiO2	Fraction of inspired oxygen
FRC	Functional residual capacity
FVC	Force vital capacity
GA	General anesthesia
HFNC	High flow nasal cannula
HH	Active humidifiers
HME	Heat and moisture exchangers
IAP	ICU-acquired pneumonia
ICU	Intensive care unit
IL	Interleukin
iMV	Invasive mechanical ventilation
IPAP	Inspiratory positive airway pressure
IR-PEP	Inspiratory resistance-positive expiratory pressure
LOS	Length of hospital stay
LV	Left ventricular
NAVA	Neurally adjusted ventilatory assist
NIV	Non-invasive mechanical ventilation
NT	N-terminal proBNP
OSA	Obstructive sleep apnea
PaO2	Partial pressure of oxygen in arterial blood

PaO2/FiO2	Partial pressure of oxygen to fraction of oxygen ratio
PEEP	Positive end-expiratory pressure
PEP	Positive expiratory pressure
pMDI	Pressurized metered dose inhalers
Pms	Mean systemic pressure
PPCs	Postoperative pulmonary complications
Pra	Right atrial pressure
PSV	Pressure support ventilation
RCT	Randomized controlled trial
SpO_2	Peripheral oxygen saturation
S/T	Spontaneous/timed
VHC	Valved holding chambers
VMN	Vibrating network nebulizer
VT	Tidal volume

Part I

Ventilatory Modes, Ventilators and Interfaces

Non-invasive Ventilation: Modes of Delivery and Interfaces

Maria Vargas and Andrea Servillo

Contents

Non-invasive ventilation (NIV) involves the application of positive pressure to help maintain ventilation in patients with compromised respiratory function [1]. The mechanism of NIV is similar to invasive positive pressure mechanical ventilation (MV). According to Mehta and Hill [2], positive pressure is delivered to the lungs to increase transpulmonary pressure on inhalation, while exhalation is controlled by elastic recoil of the alveoli and expiratory muscles. The major difference between NIV and MV is the use of interfaces. While MV involves intubation or tracheostomy, NIV delivers positive pressure through a mask (e.g., oronasal and facial). Some of the fundamental goals of NIV treatment include avoidance of intubation, decreased mortality rates, decreased incidences of ventilator-associated pneumonia (VAP), improved gas exchange, decreased ventilation time, and increased patient comfort [1].

1.1 Modes of Delivery

NIV is delivered via multiple modes, with the two most common being continuous positive airway pressure (CPAP) and bilevel positive airway pressure (BiPAP).

CPAP. This method involves the application of simultaneous inspiratory and expiratory pressure during spontaneous breathing [3]. It can be administered through endotracheal intubation or non-invasively via a facial mask or helmet. It

M. Vargas (✉)
Department of Neurosciences, Reproductive and Odontostomatological Sciences, University of Naples "Federico II", Naples, Italy
e-mail: maria.vargas@unina.it

A. Servillo
Department of Ophthalmology, University Vita-Salute, IRCCS Ospedale San Raffaele, Milan, Italy

G. Servillo, M. Vargas (eds.), *Non-invasive Mechanical Ventilation in Critical Care, Anesthesiology and Palliative Care*, https://doi.org/10.1007/978-3-031-36510-2_1

became increasingly popular in the 1980s when its success in treating obstructive sleep apnea and other chronic respiratory conditions was discovered [4]. The overall goal of CPAP is to decrease the work of breathing. CPAP is the most basic level of support and provides constant fixed positive pressure throughout inspiration and expiration, causing the airways to remain open and reduce the work of breathing [5]. This results in a higher degree of inspired oxygen than other oxygen masks. When indicated for home use, it is usually via a low flow generator and is commonly used for patients requiring nocturnal CPAP for sleep apnea [6]. High flow systems used in a hospital environment are designed to ensure that airflow rates delivered are greater than those generated by the distressed patient [6]. As well as having an effect on respiratory function, it can also assist cardiac function where patients have a low cardiac output with preexisting low blood pressure [6]. It is also commonly used for severe obstructive sleep apnea and also for type one respiratory failure, for example, acute pulmonary edema (by recruiting collapsed alveoli). *BiPAP*. Unlike CPAP, BiPAP involves the in application of two different levels of pressure: higher inspiratory pressure and lower expiratory pressure with oxygen [4]. It is administered non-invasively through a facial or nasal mask. Similar to CPAP, the patient receiving BiPAP must be able to spontaneously breathe to receive ventilation. NIV is often described as BiPAP; however, BiPAP is actually the trade name. As the name suggests, it provides differing airway pressure depending on inspiration and expiration. The inspiratory positive airways pressure (iPAP) is higher than the expiratory positive airways pressure (ePAP) [7]. The iPAP is also known as pressure support (PS). Therefore, ventilation is provided mainly by iPAP, whereas ePAP recruits under-ventilated or collapsed alveoli for gas exchange and allows for the removal of the exhaled gas.

1.2 Types of Interfaces

Unlike traditional MV, NIV is administered non-invasively through different facial interfaces. Some of these interfaces include, but are not limited to, nasal, full facial, mouthpiece, and helmet.

Nasal. As one of the initial masks used for NIV, nasal masks continue to be one of the common masks used for this treatment (Fig. 1.1c). Consisting of plastic, the nasal interface surrounds the entire nose, resting on top of the bridge of the nose [1]. It is often triangular or conical in shape. However, over time, it is reported that several complications (such as mask intolerance and air leakage) resulted from the use of this interface. Similar alternative, such as nasal pillows, helps to alleviate the discomfort often associated with the traditional nasal mask (Fig. 1.1e). Nasal pillows are soft cushions inserted into the nasal nares during treatment [2].

Full Facial. Another option instead of the nasal interface is the full facial (Fig. 1.1a). Also known as the oronasal mask, it covers from the bridge of the nose to around the mouth, while headgear and straps help to hold the mask in place. This interface is common in acute care settings to treat [2]. *Mouthpiece.* Infrequently used, mouthpieces are used during the day for ventilation (Fig. 1.1d). This interface fits into the mouth, without any irritation to the face. However, due to its placement, it is only recommended for use during the patient's waking hours. Another interface must be used while the patient is asleep to prevent aspiration [1].

Helmet. Although not approved in the United States, the helmet interface is another option (Fig. 1.1f). It encloses the patient's head into NIV therapy, resulting in less skin breakdown compared to the other interfaces. The helmet is held in place by straps attached to the axillary region [1].

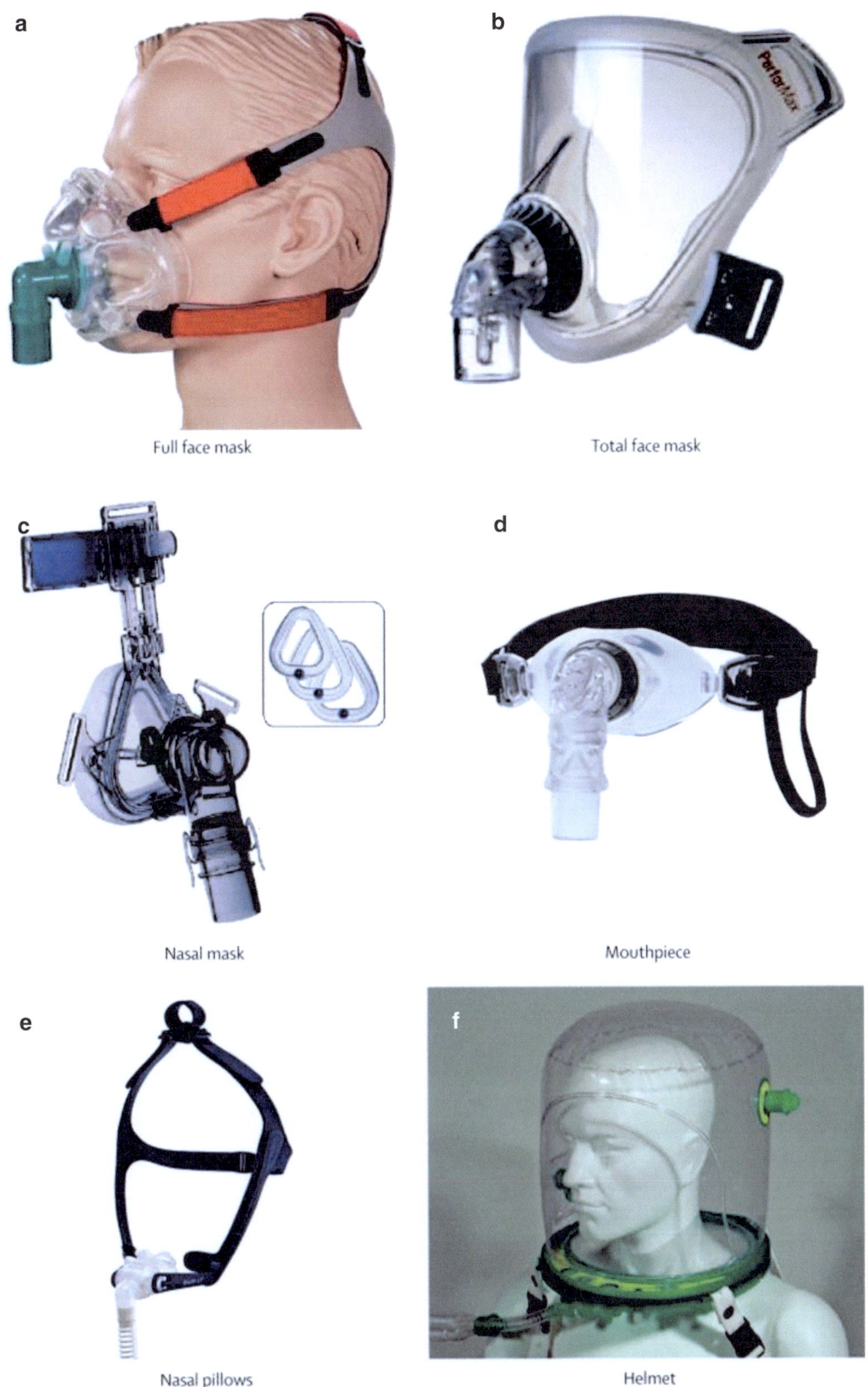

Fig. 1.1 Interfaces used during non-invasive positive pressure ventilation

1.3 Choosing the Right Non-invasive Ventilation (NIV) Interfaces

For non-invasive ventilation (NIV) to be successful, patients must adhere to the therapy you prescribe. In many cases, this has a lot to do with the mask interface that is provided for the patient. Here, we'll review the different types of mask interfaces you can choose from.

There are many varieties of masks that are used for the delivery of NIV which can be broadly categorized into nasal masks, facial masks (which can be partial or total), and helmet masks. There is no lack of ingenuity of design, as a quick internet search for NIV masks can result in dozens of varieties. Despite the myriad of options, the selection of masks in the inpatient setting is limited: the most common masks are the oronasal face mask, used in the majority of cases, followed by nasal masks, full face masks (not shown), and helmets [8]. Despite decades of research in NIV and frequent use of NIV in clinical settings, a statement published in 1994 still rings true with regard to the choice and selection of facial masks: "The optimal interface and ventilator design have not been determined, and these may differ among patients" [8].

Face masks are the most common interface used in acute respiratory failure. Due to the inspiratory demand of patients with respiratory failure, many patients utilize their mouths for inspiration to bypass nasal resistance. A face mask that covers the mouth and nose, or less commonly one that covers the mouth, nose, and eyes, can provide a comfortable fit while preventing pressure loss due to air leaking from the perimeter of the mask.

Nasal masks are most commonly used for long-term ventilation, but can also be used for acute hypoxic or hypercapnic respiratory failure. The two most common varieties are nasal masks, which cover the nose, and nasal pillows, which support tubing that inserts externally into the nares. Both types allow for eating and drinking, patients can better tolerate coughing, and

there are fewer complaints of claustrophobia with this interface.

Helmet interfaces are the least common but have recently shown the most promise with regard to NIV. They have a collar attached at the neck and shoulders and a hood that allows for gas exchange. There are two ports into the helmet—one for gas entry and one for exhalation of expired gases. A small study recently conducted in patients with acute respiratory distress syndrome (ARDS) demonstrated good outcomes in patients with helmet interface NIV.

To allow patients the greatest benefit from NIV, you may need to rotate between the different mask interfaces. Due to the pressure placed by the tight fit of an oronasal mask, allowing a break with a nasal pillow may allow for a longer duration of prescribed therapy and reduce the potential complications of skin breakdown.

References

1. Kacmarek RM. Noninvasive positive pressure ventilation. In: Wilkins RL, Stoller JK, Kacmarek RM, editors. Egan's fundamentals of respiratory care. 9th ed; 2009. p. 1091–114.
2. Mehta S, Hill NS. State of the art: noninvasive ventilation. Am J Respir Crit Care Med. 2000;163:540–77.
3. Bucher L, Seckel MA. Nursing management: critical care. In: Lewis SL, Dirksen SR, editors. Medical-surgical nursing: assessment and Management of Clinical Problems. St. Louis: Elsevier Mosby; 2011. p. 1681–716.
4. Burns S. Noninvasive positive pressure ventilation: continuous positive airway pressure (CPAP) and bilevel positive airway pressure (BiPAP). In: Wiegand DJ, editor. ACCN; 2011.
5. Nehyba K. Continuous positive airway pressure ventilation part one: physiology and patient care. Br J Card Nurs. 2006;1(12):575–9. https://doi.org/10.12968/bjca.2006.1.12.22455.
6. Nehyba K. Continuous positive airway pressure ventilation. Part two: indications and contraindications. Br J Card Nurs. 2007;2(1):18–24. https://doi.org/10.12968/bjca.2007.2.1.22638.
7. Hörmann C, Baum M, Putensen CH, Mutz NJ, Benzer H. Biphasic positive airway pressure (BIPAP) – a new mode of ventilatory support. Eur J Anaesthesiol. 1994;11(1):37–42.
8. Meyer TJ, Hill NS. Noninvasive positive pressure ventilation to treat respiratory failure. Ann Intern Med. 1994;120:760–70.

Continuous Positive Airway Pressure: High Flow CPAP

2

Carmine Iacovazzo, Claudia Veropalumbo, and Giuseppe Servillo

Contents

2.1 Continuous Positive Airway Pressure

Continuous positive airway pressure (CPAP) is a spontaneous breathing mode that takes place at an operator-determined level of positive pressure, which is maintained throughout the whole ventilatory cycle. CPAP does not actively assist ventilation: the ventilator does not cycle during CPAP and no additional pressure above the level of CPAP is provided by the breathing circuit to the patient; no mandatory breaths are delivered and it only provides patient-triggered and patient-cycled breaths.

CPAP can be provided as a standalone mode or in combination with other modes, like PSV or even Intermittent Mandatory Ventilation (IMV). It can be applied by mask, helmet, or via a cuffed endotracheal or tracheostomy tube; it may be provided through the mechanical ventilator or even using a high-flow gas source and a PEEP valve. Portable CPAP machines have also been developed for non-acute care setting and even in-home use.

The elevated airway pressure provided both during inspiration and expiration ensures respiratory muscle assistance, resulting in muscle unloading and reduction of inspiratory work of breathing (WOB); as a consequence, CPAP improves oxygenation, prevents alveolar collapse and atelectasis, and increases functional residual capacity (FRC) and the lung surface area for gas exchange.

CPAP setting requires careful hemodynamic monitoring, as the augmentation of intrathoracic pressure decreases venous return, cardiac output, and blood pressure.

C. Iacovazzo (✉) · C. Veropalumbo · G. Servillo
Department of Neuroscience and Reproductive and Odontostomatological Sciences, University of Naples Federico II, Naples, Italy

© The Author(s), under exclusive license to Springer Nature Switzerland AG 2023
G. Servillo, M. Vargas (eds.), *Non-invasive Mechanical Ventilation in Critical Care, Anesthesiology and Palliative Care*, https://doi.org/10.1007/978-3-031-36510-2_2

2.1.1 Indications

CPAP is generally the first-line treatment of Obstructive sleep apnea (OSA) both in hospital and home settings. Non-invasive CPAP delivered by oral or nasal mask at pressures in the range of 4–20 cmH_2O forces air into the upper airways to prevent soft tissues from collapsing, airway obstruction, and apnea [1]. It has been shown to be effective in reducing symptoms of sleepiness and improving the quality of life in moderate to severe OSA [2].

In the acute setting, the main goal in the use of CPAP is the avoidance of endotracheal intubation and mechanical ventilation. It is considered as a first-line strategy in the management of patients with cardiogenic pulmonary edema (CPE), as it decreases the systemic venous return and left ventricle filling pressure, limiting pulmonary edema; CPAP has been proven to decrease the need for endotracheal intubation and hospital mortality in these patients [3].

Moreover, very high levels of CPAP for brief periods of time (e.g., 40 cmH_2O for 40 s) have been suggested as a part of recruitment maneuvers to open collapsed alveoli in selected patients with ARDS.

Furthermore, the CPAP mode is frequently used to evaluate whether the patient can be weaned from the ventilator in spontaneous breathing trials, and it is also applied in the postoperative period with the aim of improving gas exchange in patients with respiratory failure or preventing atelectasis [4].

The evidence for the use of CPAP in other indications is weaker.

In the outpatient setting, adherence to CPAP is sometimes poor due to a tight-fitting mask, to frequent leaks around the interface that lead to patient–ventilator asynchronies, to positive pressure non-tolerance, and claustrophobia. Close observation and frequent reevaluation of the patient are fundamental to promptly identify CPAP failure and re-customize the ventilation strategy.

2.2 High Flow CPAP

The High Flow CPAP concept was first used in neonatal intensive care units as an alternative to standard nasal CPAP in premature neonates [5].

Regarding critically ill adults, many published reports suggest that HF-CPAP delivered by Nasal Cannula (High Flow Nasal Cannula, HFNC) decreases breathing frequency and work of breathing and reduces the need for respiratory support escalation in patients with respiratory failure with diverse underlying diseases.

The apparatus consists of an air/oxygen blender, an active heated humidifier, a single heated circuit, and a nasal cannula. HF-CPAP delivers oxygen flows of up to 60 L/min. The gas delivered to the patient is humidified and heated, while FiO_2 can easily reach more than 80%.

Usually in standard low flow oxygen therapy, oxygen is not or inadequately humidified with bubble humidifiers, and complaints, especially dry nose, dry throat, and nasal pain, are common. Insufficient heating and humidification lead to poor tolerance to oxygen therapy [6, 7].

Moreover, the nasal mucosa receptors react to cold and dry gas by stimulating a protective bronchoconstriction, while the heated, humidified air generates a beneficial effect on the ciliary movement, clearing of secretions, and prevention of atelectasis. In addition, the appropriate heating and humidification of the airways guaranteed by HF-CPAP is associated with improved pulmonary compliance and elasticity compared with dry, cold gas.

With standard oxygen, the maximal FiO_2 does not exceed 70% despite a reservoir mask and a flow rate of 15 L/min [8, 9]. In addition, the inspiratory peak flow of a patient suffering from ARF can even exceed 60 L/min in severe cases, which is greatly higher than the flow rate provided with standard oxygen: for that reason, oxygen is mixed with room air, decreasing the delivered FiO_2 to the patient [10]. The improvement in oxygenation seen with HFNC may partially be due to minimized dilution of delivered oxygen, reaching a maximal FiO_2 of more than 80%.

Furthermore, HFNC removes the air contained in the nasopharyngeal cavity, decreasing anatomic dead space and improving alveolar ventilation and CO_2 clearance [11, 12].

Although there is no pressure support in HFNC itself, the high flow enables the generation of levels of CPAP directly proportional to the delivered gas flow. The high flow continuously delivered creates a certain degree of resistance during expiration (PEEP effect), also because of the nasal obstruction guaranteed by the large nasal prongs. Consequently, the PEEP effect is markedly reduced when the patient opens the mouth. A positive linear relationship was found between the flow delivered and the airway pressure generated: for every 10 L/min increase in flow, the mean airway pressure increases by 0.69 cmH_2O in the mouth-closed position and by 0.35 cmH_2O in the mouth-open position [13].

One of the perceived benefits of HF-CPAP is the enhanced patient comfort and tolerability leading to improved compliance with the therapy [14, 15]. Tolerance of NHF has been demonstrated in several studies and is presumed to be due not only to optimal heat and humidity of gas, but also because a nasal interface lets patients eat, drink, sleep, and communicate more comfortably, without the need of removing the device [14, 16, 17]. This has led to enhanced patient comfort, fewer withdrawals of the interface, and subsequent desaturations, when compared with face mask oxygen therapy [18]. For intensive care unit (ICU) patients with ARF, it is unusual for HFNC to be interrupted by reason of discomfort [19].

2.2.1 Indications

All physiological effects and beneficial properties mentioned until now together enable breathing pattern, gas exchange, and dyspnea improvement, reduce work of breathing and respiratory rate, and guarantee a better comfort with less sensation of dryness of the upper airways. Using HFNC in clinical practice might improve the patient's outcome in some specific population and particularly in those who present to the emergency department and to the intensive care unit (ICU) [20].

Hypercapnic respiratory failure is a frequently encountered problem in those settings. The ability of HFNC to wash out dead space may reduce CO_2 rebreathing and explain its positive results in patients with hypercapnic respiratory failure. Millar et al. have reported the successful use of HFNC to handle the hypercapnic respiratory failure of patients intolerant to conventional NIV [21]. Testing *COPD* patient exercise breathing with an unloaded bicycle ergometer, Chatila et al. observed improved exercise capacity and better oxygenation with HFNC compared to spontaneous breathing [22].

HFNC has also been found to be effective for *mild to moderate hypoxemic respiratory failure.* Sztrymf et al. investigated its efficiency, safety, and outcome in ICU patients with ARF, comparing standard oxygen therapy via a face mask and HFNC. HFNC was associated with marked reductions in breathing frequency, heart rate, dyspnea score, supraclavicular retraction, and thoracoabdominal asynchrony, as well as notably increase in SpO_2, and HFNC was not stopped because of intolerance. On the other hand, HFNC has not been recommended for *severe hypoxemic respiratory failure* because of doubts about ensuring positive pharyngeal pressure [23].

Furthermore, several studies have investigated the use of NHFC post extubation to improve gas exchange, reduce respiratory rate, and improve comfort; HFNC seems to reduce the need for NIPPV and re-intubation. Maggiore et al. have compared the effects of oxygen therapy via a Venturi mask and HFNC on gas exchange and clinical outcomes. The PaO_2/FIO_2 ratio was higher with HFNC than with the Venturi mask. With HFNC, fewer patients required NPPV and re-intubation [24].

On the other hand, HF-CPAP was also tested in *pre-intubation oxygenation.*

Intubation in the ICU is often performed for hypoxemic, unstable patients and is associated with significant complications. Preoxygenation via an oxygen mask is routinely used to prevent desaturation, but severe hypoxemia may still occur. NIPPV has been shown to be more effective to reduce the incidence of desaturation; however, this technique has to be interrupted during the procedure. Because nasal cannulas do not interfere with the laryngoscopy, HFNC continuously provides a high flow rate of gas without any interruption and constant FiO_2 during the apneic period of tracheal intubation [25].

Similarly, when performing *bronchoscopy*, HFNC may be valid method for delivering oxygen in patients at risk for bronchoscopy-induced respiratory [26].

2.2.2 How to Start

When commencing HF-CPAP, once the most appropriately sized interface is been chosen, encourage patient to breathe in and out through the nose with their mouth closed. It is advisable to start with flows at a lower rate to allow the patient to get used to the sensation of heat, humidity, and flow, and then slowly increase flow to desired levels by 5 mL/min step. It may be appropriate to provide continuous monitoring of heart rate, respiratory rate, and SpO_2. Blood gas measurements should be undertaken repeatedly over time.

2.3 Conclusions

The use of HF-CPAP has increased rapidly since its introduction thanks to the spreading evidence that it is related to a number of beneficial outcomes not usually associated to standard oxygen therapies.

Additional investigations are needed in order to resolve some important issues, such as reliable indicators of success or failure, and above all, its definite indications among different patient groups.

References

1. Kushida CA, Chediak A, Berry RB, Brown LK, Gozal D, Iber C, Parthasarathy S, Quan SF, Rowley JA. Clinical guidelines for the manual titration of positive airway pressure in patients with obstructive sleep apnea. Positive airway pressure titration task force of the American Academy of sleep medicine. J Clin Sleep Med. 2008;4:157–71.
2. Evans TW, Albert RK, Angus DC, et al. International consensus conferences in intensive care medicine: noninvasive positive pressure ventilation in acute respiratory failure. Am J Respir Crit Care Med. 2001;163:283–91.
3. Bello G, De Santis P, Antonelli M. Non-invasive ventilation in cardiogenic pulmonary edema. Ann Transl Med. 2018;6(18):355. https://doi.org/10.21037/atm.2018.04.39.
4. Ireland CJ, Chapman TM, Mathew SF, Herbison GP, Zacharias M. Continuous positive airway pressure (CPAP) during the postoperative period for prevention of postoperative morbidity and mortality following major abdominal surgery. Cochrane Database Syst Rev. 2014;2014(8):CD008930. https://doi.org/10.1002/14651858.CD008930.pub2.
5. Campbell D, Shah P, Shah V, et al. Nasal continuous positive airway pressure from high flow cannula versus infant flow for preterm infants. J Perinatol. 2006;26:546–9.
6. Campbell EJ, Baker MD, Crites-Silver P. Subjective effects of humidification of oxygen for delivery by nasal cannula. A prospective study. Chest. 1988;93(2):289–93.
7. Chanques G, Contantin JM, Sauter M, Jung B, Sebbane M, Verzilli D. Discomfort associated with underhumidified high-flow oxygen therapy in critically ill patients. Intensive Care Med. 2009;35(6):996–1003. https://doi.org/10.1007/s00134-009-1456-x.
8. Frat JP, Thille AW, Mercat A, et al. High-flow oxygen through nasal cannula in acute hypoxemic respiratory failure. N Engl J Med. 2015;372(23):2185–96.
9. Sim MA, Dean P, Kinsella J, et al. Performance of oxygen delivery devices when the breathing pattern of respiratory failure is simulated. Anaesthesia. 2008;63(9):938–40. https://doi.org/10.1111/j.1365-2044.2008.05536.x.
10. Katz JA, Marks JD. Inspiratory work with and without continuous positive airway pressure in patients with acute respiratory failure. Anesthesiology. 1985;63(6):598–607. https://doi.org/10.1097/00000542-198512000-00008.
11. Ricard J-D. The high flow nasal oxygen in acute respiratory failure. Minerva Anestesiol. 2012;78(7):836–41.
12. Masclans JR, Roca O. High-flow oxygen therapy in acute respiratory failure. Clin Pulm Med. 2012;19:127–30.
13. Parke RL, Eccleston ML, SP MG. The effects of flow on airway pressure during nasal high-flow oxygen therapy. Respir Care. 2011;56(8):1151–5. https://doi.org/10.4187/respcare.01106.
14. Roca O, Riera J, Torres F, Masclans J. High-flow oxygen therapy in acute respiratory failure. Respir Care. 2010;55(4):408–13.

15. Tiruvoipati R, Lewis D, Haji K, Botha J. High-flow nasal oxygen vs high-flow face mask: a randomized crossover trial in extubated patients. J Crit Care. 2010;25(3):463–8. https://doi.org/10.1016/j.jcrc.2009.06.050.
16. Chanques G, Constantin J, Sauter M, et al. Discomfort associated with underhumidified highflow oxygen therapy in critically ill patients. Intensive Care Med. 2009;35(6):996–1003.
17. Sztrymf B, Messika J, Bertrand F, et al. Beneficial effects of humidified high flow nasal oxygen in critical care patients: a prospective pilot study. Intensive Care Med. 2011;37(11):1780–6.
18. Parke RL, SP MG, Eccleston ML. A preliminary randomized controlled trial to assess effectiveness of nasal high-flow oxygen in intensive care patients. Respir Care. 2011;56(3):265–70. https://doi.org/10.4187/respcare.00801.
19. Chikata Y, Izawa M, Okuda N, Itagaki T, Nakataki E, Onodera M, et al. Humidification performances of two high flow nasal cannula devices: a bench study. Respir Care. 2014;59(8):1186–90. https://doi.org/10.4187/respcare.02932.
20. Lenglet H, Sztrymf B, Leroy C, Brun P, Dreyfuss D, Ricard J. Humidified high flow nasal oxygen during respiratory failure in the emergency department: feasibility and efficacy. Respir Care. 2012;57(11):1873–8.
21. Millar J, Lutton S, O'Connor P. The use of high-flow nasal oxygen therapy in the management of hypercarbic respiratory failure. Ther Adv Respir Dis. 2014;8(2):63–4. https://doi.org/10.1177/1753465814521890.
22. Chatila W, Nugent T, Vance G, Gaughan J, Criner GJ. The effects of high-flow vs low-flow oxygen on exercise in advanced obstructive airways disease. Chest. 2004;126(4):1108–15. https://doi.org/10.1378/chest.126.4.1108.
23. Sztrymf B, Messika J, Bertrand F, Hurel D, Leon R, Dreyfuss D, et al. Beneficial effects of humidified high flow nasal oxygen in critical care patients: a prospective pilot study. Intensive Care Med. 2011;37(11):1780–6. https://doi.org/10.1007/s00134-011-2354-6.
24. Maggiore SM, Idone FA, Vaschetto R, Festa R, Cataldo A, Antonicelli F, et al. Nasal high-flow versus Venturi mask oxygen therapy after extubation. Am J Respir Crit Care Med. 2014;190(3):282–8. https://doi.org/10.1164/rccm.201402-0364OC.
25. Vourc'h M, Asfar P, Volteau C, et al. High-flow nasal cannula oxygen during endotracheal intubation in hypoxemic patients: a randomized controlled clinical trial. Intensive Care Med. 2015;41(9):1538–48. https://doi.org/10.1007/s00134-015-3796-z.
26. Lucangelo U, Vassallo FG, Marras E, et al. High-flow nasal interface improves oxygenation in patients undergoing bronchoscopy. Crit Care Res Pract. 2012;2012:506382. https://doi.org/10.1155/2012/506382.

High-Flow Nasal Cannula

3

Rosario Sara

Contents

3.1   Introduction

The choice of interface and ventilatory setting is crucial for the success of Non-Invasive Ventilation (NIV) for treatment in patients with acute respiratory failure. These decisions must be guided by a number of criteria such as the clinical condition, respiratory mechanics, comfort, and anthropometric characteristics of the patient [1, 2].

However, almost all the devices for NIV are responsible for various increases in respiratory dead space which in a patient on the verge of criticality can lead to a sudden worsening of gas exchanges.

Over recent years, the use of oxygen therapy through High-Flow Nasal Cannula (HFNC) in the treatment of acute hypoxemia in adults has become widespread (Fig. 3.1).

The use of this technique, despite the absence of real guidelines, has been the core of the clinical management of bronchiolitis and pediatric respiratory distress in the last decades [3].

Particularly in the post-pandemic Covid-19 era, the advantages of this method have made it one of the most used schemes in departments with higher intensity of care, up to entering international guidelines [4].

R. Sara (✉)

Department of Neuroscience and Reproductive and Odontostomatological Sciences, University of Naples Federico II, Naples, Italy

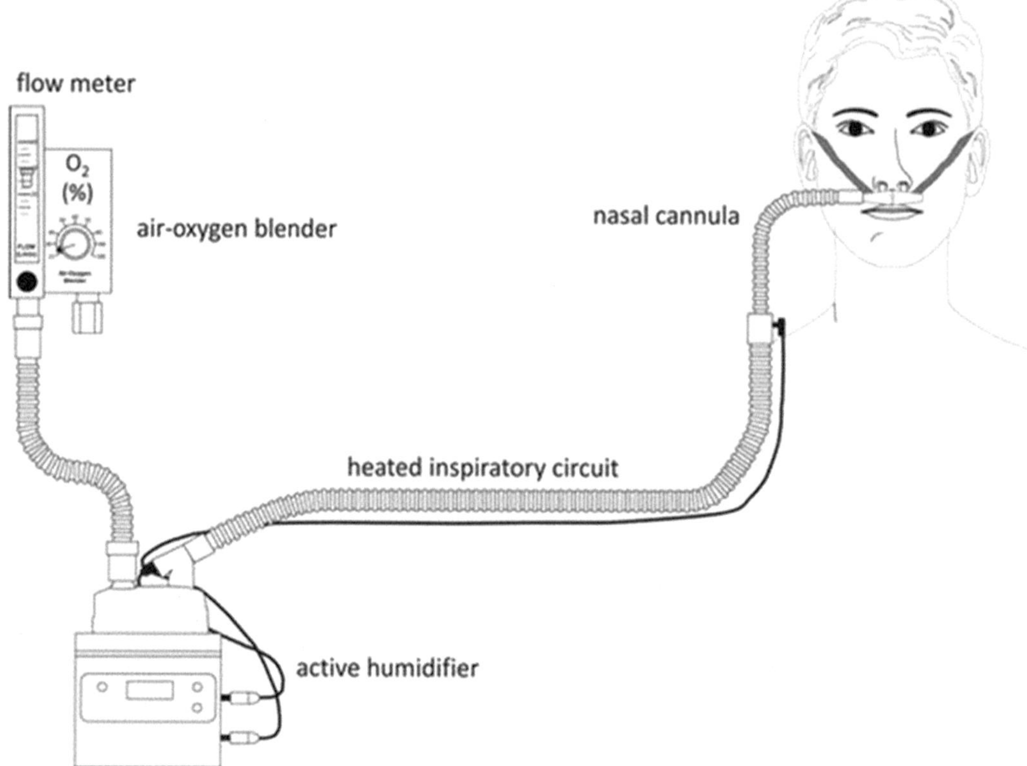

Fig. 3.1 High-flow oxygen therapy delivery system through HFNC [5]

3.2 Mechanism of Action and Clinical Benefits

The administration of oxygen via HFNC is carried out with the use of heated and humidified gas through special nasal cannulas with a larger diameter than commonly used for low flows.

A flow generator, able to get even over 60 L/min in the most recent models, is present at start of the system. It is connected to an air and oxygen mixer which allows to dispense FiO2 even by 100%. The gas mixture passes through a humidification and heating system before being convolved, through a circuit, also heated, to the patient's interface.

Then, gas mixture delivered is treated at body temperature, supersaturated with water (up to 99% relative humidity) and at a flow rate ranging from 40 to 60 L/min.

The main therapeutic effect on gas exchange is explained by the observation that the high-flow nasal delivery of O_2 makes a positive end-expiratory pressure (Peep) in the upper airways and is able to prevent the early tele-espiratory collapse of the alveolus. In this way, it also prevents what is called atelectetrauma (one of the components of the Ventilator-Induced Lung Injury, VILI) which means the alveolar barrier damage due to the continuous and complete cycle of opening and collapse of the lung unit.

The pressure level generated by the HFNC is determined by the supplied flow, the flow/body weight ratio, the ratio between the size of the nasocannula/nostrils ratio, and the opening of the mouth [6].

In addition to this effect, the presence of a high flow of gas is responsible for a reduction in respiratory resistance and respiratory dead space;

these conditions make it, together with the creation of a Peep, a recommended system for COPD patients [5].

Unlike low-flow nasal goggles, the inspiratory flow administered by the HFNC exceeds the peak of the patient's inspiratory flow, preventing the gas mixture, with preset FiO_2, from being altered by the surrounding air.

Furthermore, the administration, at the nasopharyngeal zone, of this flow higher than that carried out by the patient acts as a barrier against the expiratory flow rich in CO_2 and poor in O_2 coming from the lower respiratory tract; it is then eliminated through the mouth permitting a reduction of dead space and a further improvement of gaseous exchanges.

On the other hand, the ability to humidify and heat the gas mixture allows to preserve and increase mucociliary activity, increase patient comfort, and reduce the patient's respiratory work. The reduction of dyspnea, signs of respiratory fatigue, and respiratory rate are the first clinical signs of the efficacy of therapy with HFNC.

Finally, one of the main disadvantages of the NIV devices, such as Helmet and the Full-face mask, is the intolerability of patients for them (dry mouth and an impression of claustrophobia are the main unwanted effects reported). The patient's collaboration with the components, in addition to the ventilatory setting, represents the crossroads for the success of NIV therapy. The HFNC is placed in an intermediate position, guaranteeing, however, an excellent tolerability of the patient who can speak and feed independently.

3.3 Researches

Table 3.1 shows 19 recent large studies about HFNC in different clinical indications [7–25].

The first trials conducted on adults have shown that the use of HFNC in patients with hypoxia refractory to conventional oxygen therapy (Nasal goggles, Ventumask, etc.) led to an improvement in the mechanical aspects of respiration, to the availability of oxygen in the organism, and to the clinical condition of the patient with an average increase in the PaO_2/FiO_2 ratio [26].

In a prospective randomized trial, in which 38 critically ill patients were enrolled, the use of HFNC made it possible to avoid intubation and mechanical ventilation in 75% of cases [27]. An Italian randomized and controlled trial included 105 post-extubation patients who underwent Ventumask or HFNC and compared emogasanlitic values and clinical conditions. It highlighted how HFNC are associated with better patient comfort and a higher PaO_2/FiO_2 ratio, confirming the reduction in the use of reintubation [28],

A review of 1892 critical patients, selected from the Cochrane database, with respiratory failure found that there were no significant differences between PaO_2/FiO_2 ratio, $PaCO_2$ level, or arterial pH among patients undergoing HFNC and low-flow nasal goggles; on the other hand, he highlighted how, in patients with HFNC, there is a reduction in the average respiratory rate, in the use of intubation, and that there are no differences in mortality compared to patients undergoing NIV [29].

Table 3.1 The most recent evidence of randomized studies about high-flow nasal cannule (HFNC) in adult patients

First Author	Title (Truncated)	Number of participants	Publ. year	Type of study	Results/Recommendation
Su L	Efficacy of high-flow (…) with mild hypercapnia	202	08/2021	R	– Use of NIV or HFNC reduces intubation rate equally – HR/SpO2 is predicting factor the failure of HFNC
Ci R	Application evaluation of high-flow (…) anesthesia extubation (…)	234	08/2021	P	HFNC can effectively improve the respiratory failure of patients after extubation and reduce the occurrence of complications
Chaudhuri R	Helmet non-invasive ventilation compared to (…) high-flow nasal cannula in acute respiratory failure(…)	1345	08/2021	MR	Helmet NIV may reduce intubation rate compared to HFNC, but its effect on mortality is uncertain
Wang Y	Comparison of high-flow nasal cannula (HFNC) and conventional oxygen therapy in obese patients undergoing cardiac surgery (…)	526	08/2021	MR	For obese patients undergoing cardiac surgery, postoperative use of HFNC can maintain patient's oxygenation
Hansen CK	Characteristics (…) in COVID-19 respiratory failure: A prospective observational study	91	08/2021	P	HFNC did not result in a statistically significant difference in mortality compared to a conventional oxygen strategy
Guo K	Effects of high-flow nasal oxygen cannula versus other non-invasive ventilation in extubated patients: (…)	1746	08/2021	MR	HFNC was non-inferior to NIV in the rate of reintubation and treatment failure. And decreased the occurrence of skin lesions and post-extubation respiratory failure
Rosén J	High-flow (…) versus face mask for preoxygenation in obese patients(…)	38	07/2021	P	Face mask with PEEP was superior to HFNC for preoxygenation in obese subjects
Burra V,	A prospective (…) versus conventional nasal oxygenation following extubation of adult cardiac surgical patients	60	07/2021	P	HFNC is safe to use following extubation in adult cardiac surgical patients
Koga Y.	Association between increased nonaerated lung weight and treatment failure in patients with de novo acute respiratory failure: (…)	219	07/2021	R	Patients with a greater nonaerated lung had a higher risk of HFNC failure but not of NIV failure
Zhao Z.	Effect of non-invasive positive pressure ventilation and high-flow nasal cannula oxygen (…) of coronavirus disease 2019 patients with acute respiratory distress syndrome	41	06/2021	R	NIPPV doesn't significantly reduce the intubation rate and mortality of patients with COVID-19 accompanied with ARDS compared with HFNC

Table 3.1 (continued)

First Author	Title (Truncated)	Number of participants	Publ. year	Type of study	Results/Recommendation
Zhang P.	(…) high-flow nasal cannula oxygen therapy in post-extubation mechanically ventilated patients in intensive care unit	163 mechanical ventilation patients	06/2021	P	For patients undergoing mechanical ventilation in the ICU, HFNC after extubation can reduce the rate of weaning failure and the incidence of adverse events and the length of ICU stay
Xuan L.	Comparative study of high-flow nasal (…) in sepsis patients after weaning from mechanical ventilation in intensive care unit	283	06/2021	R	HFNC and NIV have similar efficacy in the sequential treatment of sepsis patients after weaning from MV
Garcia-Perena L.	Benefits of early use of high-flow-nasal-cannula (HFNC) in patients with COVID-19-associated pneumonia	53	06/2021	R	Early HFNC use is associated with a decrease in the need for intubation, mortality, and overall hospital stay
Deng L	Course of illness and outcomes in older COVID-19 patients treated with HFNC: a retrospective analysis	110	06/2021	R	The study suggests that the outcomes were better in severely ill elderly patients with COVID-19 receiving early compared to late HFNC
Beduneau G	Covid-19 severe hypoxemic pneumonia(…) high-flow nasal oxygen therapy as first-line management	43	06/2021	R	HFNC has first-line therapy in patients with SARS-COV-2 pneumonia, while face mask oxygen does not provide adequate respiratory support
Yu CC	High-flow nasal cannula compared (…) in the treatment of obstructive sleep apnea	28	06/2021	P	The efficacy of CPAP was superior to HFNC for both respiratory events and sleep quality
Song Y	Comparison of high-flow nasal oxygen cannula (…) hypostatic pneumonia	112	06/2021	R	FNC therapy relieves clinical symptoms more quickly than a standard oxygen mask and reduces the incidence of adverse events
Golmohamad A	(…) of high-flow nasal cannula therapy in acute hypercapnic respiratory failure—a retrospective audit	64	06/2021	R	HFNC may be an initial treatment for patients with mild acute hypercapnic respiratory failure
Rao S.	Effect of use of high-flow nasal cannula during Fiberoptic intubation under general anesthesia(…)	40	05/2021	P	HFNC were better and have beneficial effects in patients with high BMI and having a history of stridor/obstructive sleep apnea for fiberoptic intubation after muscle relaxation

P prospective, *R* retrospective, *MR* meta-analysis and review

3.4 Clinical Indications

- Acute respiratory failure (ARF) hypoxemic, mild and moderate with a PaO_2/FiO_2 ratio >100 [4]. In cases of mild ARF, the therapeutic use of HFNC is widely recognized [3]. There are no data of superiority to NIV for patients with moderate hypoxic respiratory failure. A good clinical practice suggests us to use HFNC in cases of patients with PaO_2/FiO_2 ratio <200 in a protected environment where the switch to higher ventilator supports can be quick and well-managed.
- Mild moderate hypercapnia ($PaCO_2$ <45 mmHg in restrictive pathology and <55 mmHg in obstructive); there is a lot of evidence in this regard; even though, NIV remains the gold standard for the treatment of exacerbations in COPD patients [30–33]. Patients with pH <7.2 should receive NIV or be treated with HFNC in at least sub-intensive setting.
- Do not intubate (DNT) patients, for dying patients it can be a good compromise [34].
- Postoperative or post-extubation ARF, reducing the risk of reintubation or hospitalization in the ICU and, in any case, reducing hospitalization times, risks, and costs in ICUs [28, 35].
- Obstructive Sleep Apnea Syndrome (OSAS); in patients who cannot tolerate CPAP (which is still the first choice) due to discomfort or pressure ulcers. Excellent results were obtained in OSAS patients with neurological outcomes who do not breathe well with the mouth [36, 37].
- Bronchiolitis and pediatric respiratory distress [3].
- Acute heart failure: the first data, still insufficient, underline a non-inferiority compared to NIV; however, the inaccuracy of the Peep generated represents an obstacle in these delicate patients [38]
- Chest trauma or pulmonary contusion; in these patients, the reduction in respiratory rate and the excursion of the rib cage also favor a reduction in pain.

- Pulmonary fibrosis, ensuring a chronic reduction of $PaCO_2$ [39].

3.5 Contraindications

There are no real contraindications to the use of HFNC; generally some contraindications are admitted from the use of NIV.

Patients with severe respiratory distress who already show signs of failure, with severe respiratory acidosis, tachycardia, or hemodynamically unstable (requiring high dosages of vasoactive drugs) should undergo non-invasive ventilation (NIV) or mechanical ventilation (VM) [33].

Similarly, patients in coma, with epileptic seizures or severe central neurological disorders, or otherwise unable to protect the airways and eliminate secretions, facial anthropometric alterations (congenital or post-trauma), severe gastroesophageal bleeding, or undrained pneumothorax will be excluded from trials with HFNC.

It is therefore essential to understand when inappropriate use of HFNCs is delaying the use of greater ventilatory support and to shift to it as soon as possible. A first approach to the predictive factors of HFNC failure was obtained with a retrospective study that showed that a PaO_2/FiO_2 ratio of less than 42 and almost critical clinical conditions, highlighted by an APACHE score greater than 16, can be criteria of exclusion from a cycle of HFNC, which can only dramatically delay the early use of NIV or mechanical ventilation (MV) [40].

Ultimately, close monitoring in the first hour from the initiation of oxygen therapy with HFNC of PaO_2, $PaCO_2$, serum lactate levels, and patient respiratory dynamics is essential to discriminate patients who can benefit from this therapy and avoid serious delays in switching to higher respiratory supports.

3.6 Complications

- Pneumothorax, extremely rare and especially in patients with previous severe lung diseases. In this regard, it is interesting to note that unlike CPAP it is possible to accurately monitor the strength of pressures administered, as the latter is influenced by various factors previously mentioned.

- Gastric distension, clearly reduced compared to a Full-face mask with NIV.
- Decubitus injuries caused by fasteners or related to the displacement of the cannula; particular attention should be given to neurological or DNT patients who, in the presence of a reduction in autonomy, risk greater damage to the mucous membranes and conjunctiva.
- Genesis of an autoPeep and worsening of respiratory work; possible occurrence especially in patients with functional upper airway obstructions such as OSAS patients.

3.7 HFNC in the COVID-19 Pandemic

The great interest about HNFC in recent years has reached its peak in the period of the Covid-19 pandemic.

The two determining factors for a greater use of them in patients with Sars-Cov-2 infection were a lower risk of aerosolization and environmental contamination (as patients could keep a protective mask on the mouth) and a reduction, for the same amount of Peep estimated, of the risk of VILI in already severely compromised lungs compared to patients in NIV [41].

The great interest in HNFCs in recent years has reached its peak in the period of the Covid-19 pandemic.

The two determining factors for a greater use of them in patients with Sars-Cov-2 infection were a lower risk of aerosolization and environmental contamination (as patients could keep a protective mask on the mouth) and a reduction, for the same amount of Peep estimated the risk of VILI in already severely compromised lungs compared to patients in NIV [41].

At the beginning of the pandemic, the initial data, albeit minimal, indicated non-inferiority with respect to NIV in these patients, especially in avoiding orotracheal intubation [42]. At the turn of the second wave, a multicenter review with rather stringent exclusion criteria highlighted how the use of HFNCs was useful both for the patient's clinical conditions and for reducing the risk of infections among healthcare professionals.

Patients with COVID-19 pneumonia with oxygen saturation of less than 80% and signs of respiratory muscle engagement are not eligible for the use of HFNC in place of NIV or invasive mechanical ventilation [43].

As with all diagnostic and therapeutic methods for patients with Sars-Cov-2, we are also awaiting results of greater breadth for high-flow oxygen therapy. Despite this, HFNCs represent a widely used therapeutic choice in clinical practice around the world in Covid-19 patients with mild and moderate ARDS.

Given the particular vulnerability of these patients, characterized by a rapid and intense alveolar derecruitment and an important impairment of gas exchange, a stringent selection and an even closer monitoring of the candidates to be submitted to HFNC are even more important to avoid dramatic delays in the switch to NIV or MV.

References

1. Meduri GU. Noninvasive positive-pressure ventilation in patients with acute respiratory failure. Clin Chest Med. 1996;17(3):513–53. https://doi.org/10.1016/s0272-5231(05)70330-0.
2. Meduri G, Spencer SE. Noninvasive mechanical ventilation in the acute setting. Technical aspects, monitoring and choice of interface. Eur Respir Monogr. 2001;6:106–24.
3. Wilkinson D, Andersen C, O'Donnell CP, De Paoli AG. High flow nasal cannula for respiratory support in preterm infants. Cochrane Database Syst Rev. 2011;2(2):CD006405.
4. Rochwerg B, Einav S, Chaudhuri D, et al. The role for high flow nasal cannula as a respiratory support strategy in adults: a clinical practice guideline. Intensive Care Med. 2020;46:2226–37. https://doi.org/10.1007/s00134-020-06312-y.
5. Nishimura M. High-flow nasal cannula oxygen therapy in adults. J Intensive Care. 2015;3:15. https://doi.org/10.1186/s40560-015-0084-5.

6. Papoff P, Cicchetti R, Luciani S, et al. Ossigenoterapia ad alti flussi tramite nasocannule nel bambino con insufficienza respiratoria acuta: meccanismo d'azione e indicazioni d'uso. AreaPed. 2016;17(1):35–42. https://doi.org/10.1725/2653.27226.

7. Su L, Zhao Q, Liu T, Xu Y, Li W, Zhang A. Efficacy of high-flow nasal cannula oxygen therapy in patients with mild hypercapnia. Lung. 2021;199(5):447–56. https://doi.org/10.1007/s00408-021-00472-4. Epub ahead of print

8. Ci R, Qin Y, Ci C, Zhang C, Dong S, Li M. Application evaluation of high-flow humidified oxygen in patients with respiratory failure after general anesthesia extubation for multiple injuries. J Healthc Eng. 2021;2021:1387129. https://doi.org/10.1155/2021/1387129.

9. Chaudhuri D, Jinah R, Burns KEA, Angriman F, Ferreyro B, Munshi L, Goligher E, Scales D, Cook DJ, Mauri T, Rochwerg B. Helmet non-invasive ventilation compared to facemask non-invasive ventilation and high flow nasal cannula in acute respiratory failure: a systematic review and meta-analysis. Eur Respir J. 2021;59(3):2101269. https://doi.org/10.1183/13993003.01269-2021. Epub ahead of print

10. Wang Y, Zhu J, Wang X, Liu NA, Yang Q, Luan G, Ma X, Liu J. Comparison of high-flow nasal cannula (HFNC) and conventional oxygen therapy in obese patients undergoing cardiac surgery: a systematic review and meta-analysis. In Vivo. 2021;35(5):2521–9. https://doi.org/10.21873/invivo.12533.

11. Hansen CK, Stempek S, Liesching T, Lei Y, Dargin J. Characteristics and outcomes of patients receiving high flow nasal cannula therapy prior to mechanical ventilation in COVID-19 respiratory failure: a prospective observational study. Int J Crit Illn Inj Sci. 2021;11(2):56–60. https://doi.org/10.4103/IJCIIS.IJCIIS_181_20. Epub 2021 Jun 29

12. Guo K, Liu G, Wang W, Guo G, Liu Q. Effects of high-flow nasal oxygen cannula versus other noninvasive ventilation in extubated patients: a systematic review and meta-analysis of randomized controlled trials. Expert Rev Respir Med. 2021;16(1):109–19. https://doi.org/10.1080/17476348.2021.1964363. Epub ahead of print

13. Rosén J, Frykholm P, Fors D. High-flow nasal cannula versus face mask for preoxygenation in obese patients: a randomised controlled trial. Acta Anaesthesiol Scand. 2021;65(10):1381–9. https://doi.org/10.1111/aas.13960. Epub ahead of print

14. Burra V, Putta G, Prasad SR, Manjunath V. A prospective study on use of thrive (transnasal humidified rapid insufflation ventilatory exchange) versus conventional nasal oxygenation following extubation of adult cardiac surgical patients. Ann Card Anaesth. 2021;24(3):353–7. https://doi.org/10.4103/aca.ACA_16_20.

15. Koga Y, Kaneda K, Fujii N, Tanaka R, Miyauchi T, Fujita M, Hidaka K, Tsuruta R. Association between increased nonaerated lung weight and treatment failure in patients with de novo acute respiratory failure: difference between high-flow nasal oxygen therapy and noninvasive ventilation in a multicentre retrospective study. J Crit Care. 2021;65:221–5. https://doi.org/10.1016/j.jcrc.2021.06.025. Epub ahead of print

16. Zhao Z, Cao H, Cheng Q, Li N, Zhang S, Ge Q, Shen N, Yang L, Shi W, Bai J, Meng Q, Wu C, Wang B, Li Q, Yao G. Effect of noninvasive positive pressure ventilation and high-flow nasal cannula oxygen therapy on the clinical efficacy of coronavirus disease 2019 patients with acute respiratory distress syndrome. Zhonghua Wei Zhong Bing Ji Jiu Yi Xue. 2021;33(6):708–13. https://doi.org/10.3760/cma.j.cn121430-20210104-00002. Chinese

17. Zhang P, Li Z, Jiang H, Zhou Q, Ye X, Yuan L, Wu J, Wu J, Lu W, Tao X, Jiang X. Analysis of the effect of sequential high-flow nasal canula oxygen therapy in post-extubation mechanically ventilated patients in intensive care unit. Zhonghua Wei Zhong Bing Ji Jiu Yi Xue. 2021;33(6):692–6. https://doi.org/10.3760/cma.j.cn121430-20210116-00074. Chinese

18. Xuan L, Ma J, Tao J, Zhu L, Lin S, Chen S, Pan S, Zhu D, Yi L, Zheng Y. Comparative study of high flow nasal catheter device and noninvasive positive pressure ventilation for sequential treatment in sepsis patients after weaning from mechanical ventilation in intensive care unit. Ann Palliat Med. 2021;10(6):6270–8. https://doi.org/10.21037/apm-21-8.

19. García-Pereña L, Ramos Sesma V, Tornero Divieso ML, Lluna Carrascosa A, Velasco Fuentes S, Parra-Ruiz J. Benefits of early use of high-flow-nasal-cannula (HFNC) in patients with COVID-19 associated pneumonia. Med Clin (Barc). 2021;158(11):540–2. https://doi.org/10.1016/j.medcli.2021.05.015. English, Spanish. Epub ahead of print.

20. Deng L, Lei S, Wang X, Jiang F, Lubarsky DA, Zhang L, Liu D, Han C, Zhou D, Wang Z, Sun X, Zhang Y, Cheung CW, Wang S, Xia Z, Applegate RL, Tang J, Mai Z, Liu H, Xia Z. Course of illness and outcomes in older COVID-19 patients treated with HFNC: a retrospective analysis. Aging (Albany NY). 2021;13(12):15801–14. https://doi.org/10.18632/aging.203224. Epub 2021 Jun 28

21. Beduneau G, Boyer D, Guitard PG, Gouin P, Carpentier D, Grangé S, Veber B, Girault C, Tamion F. Covid-19 severe hypoxemic pneumonia: a clinical experience using high-flow nasal oxygen therapy as first-line management. Respir Med Res. 2021;80:100834. https://doi.org/10.1016/j.resmer.2021.100834. Epub ahead of print

22. Yu CC, Huang CY, Hua CC, Wu HP. High-flow nasal cannula compared with continuous positive airway pressure in the treatment of obstructive sleep apnea. Sleep Breath. 2021;26(2):549–58. https://doi.org/10.1007/s11325-021-02413-0. Epub ahead of print

23. Song Y, Zhang J, Xing J, Wang N, Wang J. Comparison of high-flow nasal oxygen cannula therapy versus a standard oxygen face mask in patients with hypostatic pneumonia. J Int Med

Res. 2021;49(6):3000605211022279. https://doi.org/10.1177/03000605211022279.

24. Golmohamad A, Johnston R, Hay K, Tay G. Safety and efficacy of high flow nasal cannula therapy in acute hypercapnic respiratory failure - a retrospective audit. Intern Med J. 2021;52(2):259–64. https://doi.org/10.1111/imj.15400. Epub ahead of print

25. Rao S, Rai S, Das PK, Kumar S, Malviya D, Tripathi M. Effect of use of high-flow nasal cannula during fiberoptic intubation under general anesthesia: a randomized controlled trial. Anesth Essays Res. 2020;14(4):632–7. https://doi.org/10.4103/aer.aer_55_21. Epub 2021 May 27

26. Roca O, Riera J, Torres F, Masclans JR. High-flow oxygen therapy in acute respiratory failure. Respir Care. 2010;55(4):408–13.

27. Sztrymf B, Messika J, Bertrand F, Hurel D, Leon R, Dreyfuss D, Ricard JD. Beneficial effects of humidified high flow nasal oxygen in critical care patients: a prospective pilot study. Intensive Care Med. 2011;37(11):1780–6. https://doi.org/10.1007/s00134-011-2354-6. Epub 2011 Sep 27

28. Maggiore SM, Idone FA, Vaschetto R, Festa R, Cataldo A, Antonicelli F, Montini L, De Gaetano A, Navalesi P, Antonelli M. Nasal high-flow versus venturi mask oxygen therapy after extubation. Effects on oxygenation, comfort, and clinical outcome. Am J Respir Crit Care Med. 2014;190(3):282–8. https://doi.org/10.1164/rccm.201402-0364OC.

29. Ou X, Hua Y, Liu J, Gong C, Zhao W. Effect of high-flow nasal cannula oxygen therapy in adults with acute hypoxemic respiratory failure: a meta-analysis of randomized controlled trials. CMAJ. 2017;189(7):E260–7. https://doi.org/10.1503/cmaj.160570.

30. Brochard L, Mancebo J, Wysocki M, Lofaso F, Conti G, Rauss A, et al. Noninvasive ventilation for acute exacerbations of chronic obstructive pulmonary disease. N Engl J Med. 1995;333(13):817–22.

31. Ozyilmaz E, Ozsancak A, Nava S. Timing of non-invasive ventilation failure: causes, risk factors, and potential remedies. BMC Pulm Med. 2014;14:19.

32. Millar J, Lutton S, O'Connor P. The use of high-flow nasal oxygen therapy invthe management of hypercarbic respiratory failure. Ther Adv Respir Dis. 2014;8(2):63–4.

33. Ricard JD, Dib F, Esposito-Farese M, Messika J, Girault C, REVA network. Comparison of high flow nasal cannula oxygen and conventional oxygen therapy on ventilatory support duration during acute-on-chronic respiratory failure: study protocol of a multicentre, randomised, controlled trial. The 'HIGH-FLOW ACRF' study. BMJ Open. 2018;8(9):e022983. https://doi.org/10.1136/bmjopen-2018-022983.

34. Peters SG, Holets SR, Gay PC. High-flow nasal cannula therapy in do-not-intubate patients with hypoxemic respiratory distress. Respir Care. 2013;58(4):597–600. https://doi.org/10.4187/respcare.01887.

35. Rello J, Pérez M, Roca O, Poulakou G, Souto J, Laborda C, et al. High-flow nasal therapy in adults with severe acute respiratory infection. A cohort study in patients with 2009 influenza A/H1N1v. J Crit Care. 2012;27:434–9.

36. McGinley BM, Patil SP, Kirkness JP, Smith PL, Schwartz AR, Schneider H. A nasal cannula can be used to treat obstructive sleep apnea. Am J Respir Crit Care Med. 2007;176:194–200.

37. Haba-Rubio J, Andries D, Rey V, Michel P, Tafti M, Heinzer R. Effect of transnasal insufflation on sleep disordered breathing in acute stroke: a preliminary study. Sleep Breath. 2012;16:759–64.

38. Carratalá Perales JM, Llorens P, Brouzet B, Albert Jiménez AR, FernándezCañadas JM, Carbajosa Dalmau J, et al. High-flow therapy via nasal cannula in acute heart failure. Rev Esp Cardiol. 2011;64:723–5.

39. Bräunlich J, Beyer D, Mai D, Hammerschmidt S, Seyfarth H-J, Wirtz H. Effects of nasal high flow on ventilation in volunteers, COPD and idiopathic pulmonary fibrosis patients. Respiration. 2013;85:319–25.

40. Shang X, Wang Y. Comparison of outcomes of high-flow nasal cannula and noninvasive positive-pressure ventilation in patients with hypoxemia and various APACHE II scores after extubation. Ther Adv Respir Dis. 2021;15:17534666211004235. https://doi.org/10.1177/17534666211004235.

41. Li J, Fink JB, Elshafei AA, Stewart LM, Barbian HJ, Mirza SH, Al-Harthi L, Vines D, Ehrmann S. Placing a mask on COVID-19 patients during high-flow nasal cannula therapy reduces aerosol particle dispersion. ERJ Open Res. 2021;7:00519–2020. https://doi.org/10.1183/23120541.00519-2020.

42. Guy T, Créac'hcadec A, Ricordel C, Salé A, Arnouat B, Bizec JL, Langelot M, Lineau C, Marquette D, Martin F, Lederlin M, Jouneau S. High-flow nasal oxygen: a safe, efficient treatment for COVID-19 patients not in an ICU. Eur Respir J. 2020;56(5):2001154. https://doi.org/10.1183/13993003.01154-2020.

43. Agarwal A, Basmaji J, Muttalib F, Granton D, Chaudhuri D, Chetan D, Hu M, Fernando SM, Honarmand K, Bakaa L, Brar S, Rochwerg B, Adhikari NK, Lamontagne F, Murthy S, Hui DSC, Gomersall C, Mubareka S, Diaz JV, Burns KEA, Couban R, Ibrahim Q, Guyatt GH, Vandvik PO. High-flow nasal cannula for acute hypoxemic respiratory failure in patients with COVID-19: systematic reviews of effectiveness and its risks of aerosolization, dispersion, and infection transmission. Can J Anaesth. 2020;67(9):1217–48. https://doi.org/10.1007/s12630-020-01740-2. Epub 2020 Jun 15.

Humidification, Airway Secretions Management, and Aerosol Therapy

4

Giuseppe Fiorentino, Maurizia Lanza, and Anna Annunziata

Contents

G. Fiorentino (✉) · M. Lanza · A. Annunziata
Unit of Respiratory Physiopathology, Monaldi
Hospital, Naples, Italy

© The Author(s), under exclusive license to Springer Nature Switzerland AG 2023
G. Servillo, M. Vargas (eds.), *Non-invasive Mechanical Ventilation in Critical Care, Anesthesiology and Palliative Care*, https://doi.org/10.1007/978-3-031-36510-2_4

23

4.1 Introduction

4.1.1 Concept Humidity and Physiology and Role of the Upper Airway

Humidity is the amount of water vapor contained in the gas and is usually defined as absolute or relative humidity. The gas temperature is critical because its water vapor content depends on the gas temperature. The corresponding humidity is the percentage (%) of water vapor in the gas near its maximum carrying capacity. Absolute humidity is the total amount of water vapor in the gas, expressed in milligrams of suspended water in liters of gas (mg/L). Absolute humidity is directly related to the gas temperature. It is necessary in terms of humidification as, at low temperatures, the relative humidity can be 100%, while the total humidity can be far below the recommended value [1]. Inspired air conditioning occurs when a gas is heated and hydrated as it passes through the airways to reach the alveolar level in optimal conditions. Although the gas acquires temperature and humidity during its path inside the airways, the main area in which takes place the heating of the air breathed in is the nose. The temperatures of the nasal mucosa are relatively 32 °C, and although the contact time between inspired air and nasal mucosa is short, this time is sufficient to give heat. In extension, the nose has a high potential to control blood perfusion and thus balance the loss of heat during inspiration. The respiratory mucosa is lined by ciliated columnar epithelium and pseudostratified numerous goblet cells. These cells and submucosal glands support the mucosal layer that serves as a trap for the pathogens and as an interface for moisture exchange. At the level of the concluding bronchioles, the epithelium becomes a simple cubic type with minimum few goblet cells and submucosal glands. Therefore, the capacity of these pathways to perform the same level of humidification as the upper airway is limited. In addition, the air circulates through a narrow conduit by generating a turbulent flow that optimizes the heating, humidifying and filtering. The exhaled air humidity is partially preserved by

condensation on the mucosa during exhalation due to temperature differences approximately 25% of the heat and humidity increases during exhalation [2]. The eyelash movement is called metachronal ciliary; the pulse frequency is directly proportional to the temperature (t°). It is expected that at 37 °C it is 750 b/min, but at 40 C rise at 1100 b/min. Excessive moisture affects the ciliary function since it increases the volume of secretions due to its low viscosity and the risk of atelectasis obstructing the airway. This explains why at a temperature higher than 37 °C and 100% of the gas saturation it produces a gas condensation, thus causing a reduction in mucus viscosity and an increase in the pericellular liquid thickness, which may be too liquid to be adequately coupled to the tips of the eyelashes, thereby influencing the mucociliary transport. Considering the temperature of the inspired air rises throughout its passage through the airway, at the level of the alveolar-capillary interface, it is at body temperature (37 °C), with 100% relative humidity and 44 mg/L absolute humidity. The feature where the gas acquires these conditions is the isothermal saturation limit; this limit is ordinarily close to the fourth or fifth bronchial generation. It is crucial to reach the isothermal saturation limit to bypass injury to the mucosa and the ciliary epithelium. An artificial airway prevents inspired air from contacting the mucosa of the upper airway affecting conditioning gas. The normal physiology of conditioning gas is altered when the patient requires an artificial airway; intubation eliminates the natural filtration mechanisms, humidification, and warming of inspired air. The humidification of inspired gas is necessary for all mechanically ventilated patients; however, the discussion about the fitting humidification continues today [3].

NIMV provides dry and cold gas through the upper airway, causing dryness of the mucosa and respiratory dysfunction. Leakage compensation used by NIMV creates high flow during the respiratory cycle, which provides to the lack of heat and humidity [4]. Although in NIMV the upper airway is saved, humidification during NIMV might not be optimal due to the higher flow delivered, thus producing increased mucous viscosity and secretion recognition. These conditions improve the danger of obstruction of the upper airways.

4.2 Humidification Devices

Two prototypes of devices for conditioning inspired gases in the presence or inadequacy of an artificial airway are possible: heat and moisture exchangers (HME) and active humidifiers (HH) [5].

Although whichever device is chosen, it should infallibly coincide the minimum conditions to reinstate the role of the upper airway, which, according to the American Association for Respiratory Care, are [1]:

- 30 mg/L absolute humidity, 34 °C and 100% related humidity for HME.
- Within 33 mg/L and 44 mg/L absolute humidity; between 34 °C and 41 °C; 100% relative humidity for HH.

4.3 Active Humidifiers

The active humidifiers are devices formed of an electric heater placed at a plastic casing with a metal base in which is stored sterile water. When the base is heated, the water temperature rises by convection. Some active humidifiers are self-regulated by a mechanism consisting of a heating wire (a wire heated breathing circuit) that keeps constant the temperature of the gas during its passage in the circuit and a wire with two temperature sensors connected to the output of the heater (distal) and to a part of the circuit (near the patient) to control the system temperature.

4.4 Assembly

Active humidifiers are positioned in line in the inspiratory leg of the respirator. The circuit leaving the inhalation valve is connected to the inlet hole of the plastic casing, which must always be filled to the level indicated by the manufacturer.

Subsequently, a second section of the circuit (of standard length) is connected to the outlet hole of the casing and to the "Y" of the circuit responsible for supplying gas to the patient. With this type of humidification device, it is necessary to use siphons, tanks with unidirectional circulation systems that allow the excess condensate to be deposited without air leaks. Among other problems, excessive accumulation of water in the circuit can lead to self-activation, misreading of the ventilator monitor, or even the drainage of contaminated material into the patient's airways. The active humidifiers are placed in line in the inspiratory leg of the respirator. The output circuit from the inhalation valve is connected to the casing inlet hole in plastic, which must always be filled to the level indicated by the manufacturer. Subsequently, a second section of the standard length circuit is connected to the casing output hole and the "Y" of the charge circuit to provide gas to the patient. With this type of humidification device, it is required to use siphons, tanks with unidirectional circulation systems, that deposit the excess condensate without air leakage. Among other problems, the excessive accumulation of water in the circuit can lead to auto trigger, the misreading of the fan, or even to monitor drainage of contaminated material in the patient's airway. These humidifier varieties are separated into several categories: bubble humidifiers, humidifiers waterfall, bypass humidifiers, and humidifiers shirt [6]. Of the active humidification systems, the bypass is the most generally used now in the ICU; they are utilized in mechanical ventilation and non-invasive ventilation. The gas that goes to the patient moves across the heated water surface, which creates the humidification to come close to 100% RH and can deliver up to 44 mg/L of AH [7]. The water is heated via heating base, which transfers heat by convection from the metal of the bases. It is self-regulating by a servomechanism and consists of a heating cable (which controls the temperature of the gas in the circuit, thus limiting condensation in the piping and the possibility of bacterial colonization), a cable with two temperature sensors, which are secured at the output of the humidifier, and a Y-piece (near the patient) to servo-control the temperature of the system. In most current devices, the temperature is preset at 37 °C. This system manages control of the gas temperature to the patient, despite differences in the gas flow or water level in the reservoir, notwithstanding having an average time of reaction. The water that condenses the pipes is supposedly contaminated and should not be returned to the humidifier. The main obstacle with this device is that it does not filter particles [8].

4.5 Precautions and Monitoring for Active Humidifiers

- Recognize that the tubing drains the water downwards and not near the artificial airway or the ventilator.
- Place the water traps accurately to receive drained water.
- Regularly monitor the active humidifier device (water level, temperature level, indicate the presence of condensation).
- Never fill above the suggested level.
- Comply with the manufacturer's terms.
- Do not remove the condensation toward the humidifier chamber.

4.6 Passive Humidifiers

They are economical and simple to use with conventional connectors for IMV. They include a high communication surface of paper, with compressed metallic parts which attract particles of expired water vapor and heat, pressing and releasing it in the next inspiration. In daily use there are heat and moisture exchanger (HME) humidification systems, any with a particle filter. To fulfill this purpose, the HME can be Hydrophobic (HMEF, Heat-and-Moisture Exchanger Filter), Hygroscopic (HHME, Hygroscopic Heat-and-Moisture Exchanger), or both with filter (HHMEF, hygroscopic Heat-and-Moisture Exchanger and filter). Hygroscopic is an attribute of a compound chemical material, which absorbs condensation from the air. The aluminum element of this device that immediately exchanges temperatures during expiration condensation is created between the layers of this

material. The preserved heat and moisture are replaced during inspiration. Adding a fibrous component helps retain moisture and decreases the accumulation of condensation in the secondary position of the device. Hydrophobic is an adjunct for those substances or elements that resist water and cannot combine or absorb. They utilize a paper or polypropylene treated with calcium or lithium chloride, to improve moisture maintenance and repel water that is not absorbed. It is essential to consider that these devices additionally perform as a bacterial filter. The HME are situated between the Y-piece of the patient, which can increase the resistance to airflow, not only during inspiration, but also when expiration. The minimum resistance to the flow is 0.5–3.6 cm H2O/L/s. It is essential to record the dead space produced by these devices, which can be mutable. Among separate devices, according to some measurements, it can reach 95 mL. Passive humidifiers should never be used in conjunction with active humidifiers [9].

4.7 Dead Space

The working system of passive humidifiers means that a higher volume of condenser material will produce better device performance. For this reason, the 'ideal' dead space for a humidifier is approximately 50 mL. This dead space does not describe a problem for patients with invasive mechanical ventilation (iMV) because the dead space can be counterbalanced for the ventilator's programming. However, in patients with artificial airways, without the necessity of iMV, the increase in the ventilatory minute volume as a compensatory mechanism for the dead space could generate a hard-to-tolerate load in patients with low ventilatory reserve. Consequently, passive humidifiers with a small volume were produced. Although they can be more tolerable, they produce a low humidification capacity that worsens when the tidal volume (VT) increases and supplementary O2 [10]. The necessary dead space added by the passive humidifiers during iMV becomes essential when the pathology requires strategies for lung protection (low VT). Studies conducted by Prat [11] and Hinkson [12] account for this, showing significant changes in arterial carbon dioxide partial pressure (PaCO2) (and in pH) under these circumstances.

4.8 Resistance

Although the resistance of an additional device could be judged negligible (5 cmH2O/L/s assessed as dry), resistance can vary under differences in the conditions (presence of condensation, impaction due to secretions, changes in ventilatory parameters, increases in the VT and the flow). Although some studies [13] have registered that the presence of humidity in a device does not lead to essential changes in resistance, redundant condensation or impaction (due to secretions or blood) can alter it.

4.9 Active or Passive Humidification

In utilizing NIMV, the type of ventilators assumes a vital role in the decision of the humidifier to be used. For a single branch turbine ventilator and with leakage compensation, the indication for the use of HH would be in common use in patients who use non-invasive mechanical ventilation times close to 24 hours a day for the underlying clinical problems to enhance the feeling of oral dehydration and tolerance as recommended by Oto in 2014 [4]. It is also essential to examine the testimonials of Esquinas et al. [14] in terms of the factors involved in choosing the type of humidification to use, such as air leakage, interface type, type of ventilator, ambient temperature, and inhaled gas temperature between others. Considering when using HME in single-branch NIMV, there must be a description of where the exhalatory port is in the system. Current recommendations favor the use of heated humidifiers (HH) during NIMV [15], decreasing nasal resistance, helping expectoration, and increasing adhesion and comfort, especially in patients with bronchial secretions [15]. HME is not supported in NIMV because the dead space of the device harms CO2 removal and minute ventilation in patients managed with NIMV in ICU; this is more evident in hypercapnic patients [15]. *Also,* there has been seen that it increases work in breathing. In Table 4.1 are reported the main advantages and disadvantages on 'use of HME and HH'.

Table 4.1 Advantage and disadvantage of HH and HME

Devices	Advantages	Disadvantages
Active	Universal application	Cost
	Reliability	Using water
	Alarms	Condensation
	Wide ranges of temperature and humidity	Risk of contamination
	Temperature monitoring	Low possibility of electrical shock and burns
	Reaches the maximum absolute humidity	No filter
Passive	Cost	Does not apply all patients
	Passive operation	Increase dead space
	User-friendly	Increase resistance
	Removal of condensation	Potential occlusion
	Portable	Misting problems

4.10 Background Aerosol Therapy

The drug concentrations in lung tissue are affected by the aerosol dose administered, patient factors, device factors, and drug formulation. The productiveness of the aerosolized drug depends on the dose accumulated at the target site of action and its distribution in the lungs.

The overall efficiency of the aerosol system is a compound of the emitted dose (ED), the dose delivered to the lung (PSF as a surrogate marker), and lung bioavailability. The ED and the PSF are generally determined in vitro and are regulated by the characteristics of the particles and the composition of the device. The bioavailability of the drug is influenced by patient factors, such as the anatomy of the airways and lungs, the permeability of the drug through the membranes, the drug metabolism, and clearance of phagocytes in the lung [16]. We know that the air flow is not homogeneous in all lungs, even in health. The apical portions of the lungs receive a lung deposition of the order of a 2:1 ratio higher than the basal regions. This difference is significantly decreased in the supine position. Among the factors that affect the administration of aerosolized drugs in critically ill patients include: the position of the patient, the formulation, the temperature, the size of the endotracheal tube, the obstruction of the airways or the ventilatory asynchrony, the flow pattern, respiratory rate, the dose and the applied frequency, or the nebulizer position in the circuit.

4.11 Fundamentals of Aerosol Therapy

The size of the drug particles (measured in microns) used in an aerosol for respiratory diseases determines in which the airways will be deposited. The ideal size of the particles for respiratory drugs is from 1 to 8 μm. At these dimensions, the particles can reach the walls of the distal airways via sedimentation and diffusion. In contrast, the microscopic particles of the drug (<1 μm) have a poor transportability and high probability of being exhale. In contrast, very large particles (>8 μm) tend to agglomerate and settle rapidly in the upper airways (oropharynx and language), from where they can be swallowed and absorbed, finally causing systemic side effects. It should be noted that the nebulizers, devices that generate aerosols of drugs, do not allow a uniform particle size; instead, they produce a wide range of particle sizes.

The pressurized metered dose inhalers (pMDI) with valved holding chambers (VHC) have demonstrated superior deposition compared to nebulizers in various studies. However, VHC cannot be used for mechanical ventilators because of their inability to activate the device. The PPE have no fuel, they are inherently synchronized/activated with the breath, and produce small variations in particle size. The deposition in the airways may occur by inertial impaction, gravitational settling, or diffusion (Brownian motion). Due to the turbulence and high air velocities associated with aerosol, the inertial impact method is predominant in the first ten ramifications of the airways. However, in five to six generations, distal airway predominates sedimentation due to the lower air velocity [16]. At the alveolar level, a minimum air velocity means that there will be no effect of impact. A combination of sedimentation and diffusion will affect the deposition of the drug. The inspiratory flow of the patient influences the amount and type of deposited particles and the deposition mechanism. The scope of preferred aerosol is from 30 L/min to 60 L/min. Flows inspiratory elevated (>100 L/min) favor the deposition to provide high impact and penetration speed. On the contrary, low inspiratory flow (<30 L/min) favored the sedimentation, but involved the risk that the patient inhales only a tiny amount of the drug. The deposition of particles in the lower airways of children is hampered by the combination of high flow rates and decreasing diameter (from top to bottom) of the airways. The affinity of the particles for the water determines the extent to which they can change the size. For the aerosol to be successful you must consider the aerosol system. The aerosol system includes the drug, the aerosol device, the disease (which is the target site), and the patient's respiratory system. The ventilator is an additional factor in mechanically ventilated patients.

4.12   Device Effects

Nebulizers are several devices that are used to transform liquid formulations and suspensions in the form of aerosols. These devices can be used to produce larger volumes of a drug in aerosol form, intermittently or continuously, to the purpose of prevention or treatment. Depending on their development mechanism, there are three types of nebulizers: jet, ultrasonic, and SMN. The subsequent development of "new generation" devices such as the ultrasonic nebulizer and vibrating network nebulizer (VMN) has encouraged further studies and applications of aerosol therapy in the ICU because of the ability of these devices to constantly generate the particle size of aerosol desired, which is considered to be optimal for deep lung penetration. The jet nebulizers are the cheapest and simple, although they are inefficient in administering drugs. Their disadvantages are the noise, the lack of control of the dosage, and the need to modify the ventilator settings such as the airflow and the tidal volume. The ultrasonic nebulizers are rarely used and also have limitations. They are expensive, large in size, increase the concentration of the drug during nebulization, and can cause thermal inactivation of the nebulized drug. A significant fraction of the aerosolized drug is trapped in the mucous membranes of the conducting airways. Conditions such as pneumonia and other inflammatory lung diseases cause lung surfactant deficiencies in both content and effect. Drugs with high solubility are likely to have a uniform dispersion than insoluble drugs. Inferential, soluble drugs are likely to have longer and more effective lung residence times, thereby improving drug potency. Surfactant deficiency is associated with atelectasis, which in turn reduces drug deposition [17]. Where possible, pMDI with spacers should be used. The use of PPE is likely to be limited in the ICU. The device should be selected for nebuliz-

ers based on the formulation used and the desired deposition site and effect. The rate and extent of absorption of aerosolized substances depend on molecular weight, pH, electric charge, solubility, and stability.

4.13   The Heliox Effect

A mixture of helium and oxygen (heliox) reduces the density of the gas and increases the deposition of aerosols, in particular in the peripheral lung. With pMDI, it was reported that it increases Heliox administration of aerosolized medications during mechanical ventilation [18]. However, with the jet nebulizers, Heliox also increases the nebulization time, requiring higher gas flows to compensate for the low-density gas.

4.14   Type of Aerosol Generator in the Circuit

Currently, nebulizers and pMDIs, with and without spacers, are two types of devices prepared for use in mechanically ventilated patients. Depending on the site of action, they should be used in devices that produce one of the appropriate particle sizes. Nebulizers take much longer to deliver a standard dose compared to other devices. There is also a variation of efficiency between the nebulizer types and between different batches in nebulizers. This effect is accentuated if associated with the impact of different modes of ventilation and pulmonary mechanics. Meticulous cleaning and disinfection of the nebulization system can ensure a reduced risk of possible nosocomial pneumonia. The pMDI are easy to administer, require less time for staff, provide a reliable dosage, and have a minimum of bacterial contamination risk than nebulizers. When used with a collapsible spacer into the circuit, it is not necessary to disconnect the circuit. The pMDI are also cheaper nebulizers. Additionally, the location represents that the best one for the aerosol generator can be 15 cm from the Y-piece into the inspiratory, although necessary in vivo studies to draw definitive conclusions [19].

Humidification is believed to have a significant effect on aerosol drug delivery. Due to the hygroscopic effects of humidification, there may be a 2–3 times growth in particle size as they pass through the airways. This increase in size can reduce drug deposition in the peripheral lungs and hence pharmacological efficacy. The particulate air filter in the expiratory tract protects the ventilator and the flowmeter may become saturated, causing the airflow to be blocked. It is supported to replace the filter after each nebulization treatment.

4.15 Features of Breath

The aspects of the ventilator breath have an influential effect on the efficacy of the administration of aerosol. Inspiratory flows slower, inspiratory time-consuming, and tidal volumes>500 mL (using a pMDI) correlate well with improved aerosol dispensing. The common effective mixture of tidal volume, flow, and other parameters of the fan for the aerosol dispensing can be calibrated on the drug and on the dispensing device using in vitro models [20].

The positive end-expiratory pressure (PEEP) is a setting of usually used ventilation as part of the lung protective ventilation strategy in severe lung disease. PEEP has significant effects on regional ventilation and perfusion and may affect the pharmacokinetics of aerosolized medication. In an animal model that used radiotracers, it was discovered that the PEEP improves the aerosol removal [20]. This could be due to the alveolar epithelium stretching and improving the aerosol distribution in the bloodstream. Meaning: PEEP is potentially advantageous, although further data to quantify the effect on the administration of aerosolized medications are necessary.

Optimization of ventilator parameters required for antibiotic aerosol modified by Lu et al. [21]:

- Positioning of the nebulizer: in the inspiratory limb 10 cm proximal to the Y fitting.
- Diluted in 10 mL of physiological solution.
- Remove the HME filter.

- Ventilation mode—volume control.
- Airflow pattern: constant inspiratory flow.
- Ventilator settings: RR 12/min, 50% I: E ratio, VT 8 mL/kg.
- End of inspiration pause, 20% duty cycle.
- Expired aerosol particles collected in a filter.

4.16 Dose Effect and the Time

Despite the administration of inhaled medicines, significant extrapulmonary drug losses can mean that the actual amount of drug delivered may be less than the set. The doses should be different in patients with colonization, tracheobronchitis, or pneumonia. Increasing doses require longer nebulization times that are not well tolerated by patients with ARDS or other serious lung diseases. Most of the loss of drug occurs in the expiratory phase of ventilation. To minimize this loss, the activation of the inhaler or nebulizer may be coupled to inhalation.

4.17 High Flow Nasal Cannula Effect

High-flow nasal oxygen therapy is growing and generally prevalent in *intensive care* unit (ICU). A number of factors influence nebulization therapy in patients using high flow, which has recently been studied in an in vitro model [22].

1. Nebulizer Location—A location away from the humidifier (closer to the patient) improves drug delivery upstream.
2. Nebulizer type: VMNs have demonstrated better delivery than jet nebulizers, although the choice of nebulizer depends on the formulation and desired site of action.
3. Airflow: Breathing mass delivery is lower with higher airflow and improves with lower airflow.
4. Patient Efforts: Talking about the effect of airflow with a high-flow oxygen system, in situations mimicking respiratory distress (i.e., an increase in the patient's inspiratory airflow)

delivery was indeed best. An open mouth, in contrast, had no significant differences from a closed mouth with respect to drug administration.

4.18 Contemporary Applications of Aerosol Therapy in Critical Care: Focus on Antibiotics

Despite these developments, the best evidence for the administration is not enforced, particularly for aerosolized antibiotics. Data from clinical and experimental studies to aminoglycosides and colistin are perhaps the most numerous to antibiotics in intensive care. The aminoglycosides are concentration-dependent antibiotics for which the Cmax/MIC ratio describes the most of the bactericidal effect. Studies have shown that aminoglycosides intravenously penetrate evil in the epithelial lining fluid [23].

In a model of pneumonia inoculation of Escherichia coli, it was observed that the aerosolized amikacin lung reaches significant concentrations.

On the other hand, there was no accumulation effect with repeated administration and therefore no toxicity problem with the aerosolized amikacin. In experimental studies, serum concentrations of amikacin were higher when the aerosolized amikacin was used in a pneumonia model compared to healthy lungs. In addition, a combination of intravenous aminoglycosides and aerosols has not been shown to increase cure rates compared to only aerosol antibiotics [24]. Therefore, for the treatment of ventilator-associated pneumonia, aerosol therapy alone may be adequate without the need for an intravenous therapy, decreasing the risk of systemic toxicity.

4.19 Limits of Aerosol Therapy in Intensive Care

In fact, there is the possibility of causing systemic toxicity (e.g., aminoglycoside nephrotoxicity) or local toxicity in the form of irritation of the airways, cough and often bronchospasm, worsening hypoxemia (and secondary arrhythmias), and lung lesions during the use of aerosol therapy [25]. There have been reports of the fan malfunctions and obstruction of expiratory filters, contraindicated for use of drugs with lipid components or sugar lactose in the formulation (such as zanamivir or formulations of amphotericin lipid-based). You need close monitoring of the potential increase in airway pressure and oxygen saturation to anticipate serious adverse events. Tolerance aerosol is different when medications are nebulized for various periods of time. This may limit the use of the aerosol in patients with ARDS or severe hypoxemia, such as severe pneumonia (in contrast with the ventilator-associated tracheobronchitis), which often have poor tolerance [26]. The environmental contamination caused by aerosols of drugs in an open-loop system represents a small but significant risk to health care workers. The use of expiratory filters with valves in the aerosol dispensing devices could minimize this problem. This exposure to the occupational hazard should be evaluated and interventions should be implemented to mitigate the risks. When using aerosolized antibiotics, it is recommended to change the filter after each therapy.

4.20 Conclusion

During NIMV an inadequate gas conditioning has been associated with anatomical and functional impairment of the nasal mucosa. It suggests the use of active humidification (evidence 2B), while it is not recommended to use passive humidification (evidence 2C). However, recent publications using ICU ventilators disagree with these recommendations. We believe that to choose the type of humidifier for use during NIMV, there are certain aspects that must be taken into consideration as the fan type, the type of interface and losses, among others, which could favor the use of HH compared HME to improve tolerance and patient comfort. Aerosol drug delivery in NIV is affected by several factors, including type of ventilator, mode of ventilation, circuit conditions, type of interface, type of aerosol generator, breathing parameters, drug-related factors, and patient-related factors. Aerosol drug delivery during NIV has gained popularity over the years. Due to many factors that impact drug delivery to patients receiving NIV, aerosol therapy in this patient population can be extremely complex. However, if clinicians know what to use, how to use it, and why, aerosol therapy can be feasible and effective during NIV.

Conflict of Interest Author declare no interest conflict.

References

1. Restrepo RD, Walsh BK. Humidification during invasive and noninvasive mechanical ventilation: 2012. American association for respiratory care. Respir Care. 2012;57(5):782–8.
2. Keck T, Leiacker R, Heinrich A, et al. Humidity and temperature profile in the nasal cavity. Rhinology. 2000;38(4):167–71.
3. Gross JL, Park GR. Review humidification of inspired gases during mechanical ventilation. Minerva Anestesiol. 2012;78(4):496–502.
4. Oto J, Nakataki E, Okuda N, et al. Hygrometric properties of inspired gas and oral dryness in patients with acute respiratory failure during noninvasive ventilation. Respir Care. 2014;59(1):39–45.
5. Uchiyama A, Yoshida T, Yamanaka H, et al. Estimation of tracheal pressure and imposed expiratory work of breathing by the endotracheal tube, heat and moisture exchanger, and ventilator during mechanical ventilation. Respir Care. 2013;58(7):1157–69.
6. Al Ashry HS, Modrykamien AM. Review humidification during mechanical ventilation in the adult patient. Biomed Res Int. 2014;2014:715434.
7. Schena E, Saccomandi P, Cappelli S, et al. Mechanical ventilation with heated humidifiers: measurements of condensed water mass within the breathing circuit according to ventilatory setting. Physiol Meas. 2013;34(7):813–21.
8. Nishida T, Nishimura M, Fujino Y, et al. Performance of heated humidifiers with a heated wire according to ventilatory settings. J Aerosol Med. 2001. Spring;14(1):43–51.
9. Branson RD. Review humidification of respired gases during mechanical ventilation: mechanical considerations. Respir Care Clin N Am. 2006;12(2):253–61.
10. Brusasco C, Corradi F, Vargas M, et al. In vitro evaluation of heat and moisture exchangers designed for spontaneously breathing tracheostomized patients. Respir Care. 2013;58(11):1878–85.
11. Prat G, Renault A, Tonnelier JM, et al. Influence of the humidification device during acute respiratory distress syndrome. Intensive Care Med. 2003;29(12):2211–5.
12. Hinkson CR, Benson MS, Stephens LM, et al. The effects of apparatus dead space on P(aCO2) in patients receiving lung-protective ventilation. Respir Care. 2006;51(10):1140–4.
13. Lucato JJ, Tucci MR, Schettino GP, et al. Evaluation of resistance in 8 different heat-and-moisture exchangers: effects of saturation and flow rate/profile. Respir Care. 2005;50(5):636–43.
14. Esquinas Rodriguez AM, Scala R, Soroksky A, et al. Review clinical review: humidifiers during non-invasive ventilation--key topics and practical implications. Crit Care. 2012;16(1):203.
15. Mas A, Masip J. Review noninvasive ventilation in acute respiratory failure. Int J Chron Obstruct Pulmon Dis. 2014;9:837–52.
16. Laube BL, Janssens HM, de Jongh FH, et al. What the pulmonary specialist should know about the new inhalation therapies. European respiratory society., International society for aerosols in medicine. Eur Respir J. 2011;37(6):1308–31.
17. Ari A, Fink JB. Review guidelines for aerosol devices in infants, children and adults: which to choose, why and how to achieve effective aerosol therapy. Expert Rev Respir Med. 2011;5(4):561–72.
18. Goode ML, Fink JB, Dhand R, et al. Improvement in aerosol delivery with helium-oxygen mixtures during mechanical ventilation. Am J Respir Crit Care Med. 2001;163(1):109–14.
19. Dugernier J, Wittebole X, Roeseler J, et al. Influence of inspiratory flow pattern and nebulizer position on aerosol delivery with a vibrating-mesh nebulizer during invasive mechanical ventilation: an in vitro analysis. J Aerosol Med Pulm Drug Deliv. 2015;28(3):229–36.
20. Bayat S, Porra L, Albu G, et al. Effect of positive end-expiratory pressure on regional ventilation distribution during mechanical ventilation after surfactant depletion. Anesthesiology. 2013;119(1):89–100.
21. Lu Q, Luo R, Bodin L, et al. Efficacy of high-dose nebulized colistin in ventilator-associated pneumonia caused by multidrug-resistant Pseudomonas aeruginosa and Acinetobacter baumannii. Anesthesiology. 2012;117(6):1335–47.
22. Réminiac F, Vecellio L, Heuzé-Vourc'h N, et al. Aerosol therapy in adults receiving high flow nasal cannula oxygen therapy. J Aerosol Med Pulm Drug Deliv. 2016;29(2):134–41.
23. Solé-Lleonart C, Rouby JJ, Chastre J, et al. Intratracheal administration of antimicrobial agents in mechanically ventilated adults: an international survey on delivery practices and safety. Respir Care. 2016;61(8):1008–14.

24. Goldstein I, Wallet F, Nicolas-Robin A, et al. Lung deposition and efficiency of nebulized amikacin during Escherichia coli pneumonia in ventilated piglets. Am J Respir Crit Care Med. 2002;166(10):1375–81.
25. Van Heerden PV, Caterina P, Filion P, et al. Pulmonary toxicity of inhaled aerosolized prostacyclin therapy -an observational study. Anaesth Intensive Care. 2000;28(2):161–6.
26. Lu Q, Yang J, Liu Z, Gutierrez C, Aymard G, Rouby JJ. Nebulized antibiotics study group nebulized ceftazidime and amikacin in ventilator-associated pneumonia caused by Pseudomonas aeruginosa. Am J Respir Crit Care Med. 2011;184(1):106–15.

Why and When to Start Non-invasive Ventilation

5

Greta Zunino, Denise Battaglini, Patricia R. M. Rocco, and Paolo Pelosi

Contents

G. Zunino · P. Pelosi
Anesthesia and Intensive Care, San Martino
Policlinico Hospital, IRCCS for Oncology and
Neuroscience, Genoa, Italy

Department of Surgical Sciences and Integrated
Diagnostics, University of Genoa, Genoa, Italy

D. Battaglini (✉)
Anesthesia and Intensive Care, San Martino
Policlinico Hospital, IRCCS for Oncology and
Neuroscience, Genoa, Italy

Department of Medicine, University of Barcelona,
Barcelona, Spain

P. R. M. Rocco
Laboratory of Pulmonary Investigation, Carlos
Chagas Filho Biophysics Institute, Federal University
of Rio de Janeiro, Rio de Janeiro, Brazil

© The Author(s), under exclusive license to Springer Nature Switzerland AG 2023
G. Servillo, M. Vargas (eds.), *Non-invasive Mechanical Ventilation in Critical Care, Anesthesiology
and Palliative Care*, https://doi.org/10.1007/978-3-031-36510-2_5

5.1 Introduction

Non-invasive ventilation (NIV) refers to a ventilator modality that provides ventilatory support through the natural airways in a collaborating patient without the use of an invasive interface such as an endotracheal tube, laryngeal mask, or tracheostomy tube. The purpose of NIV is to give good quality ventilatory support to improve gas exchange, reduce the work of breathing, and dyspnea [1, 2].

NIV delays the possible start of invasive mechanical ventilation (IMV) and its related complications such as those associated with the loss of the protective airway reflexes, the increased risk of ventilator-associated pneumonia, the risks related to the endotracheal tube removal, and the possible occurrence of ventilator-associated lung injury (VILI) [3]. However, the use of a non-invasive interface is not exempted from complications [4, 5].

The first report regarding the use of NIV dates back to the 1940s with the iron lung used during the polio epidemic. The application of an alternate external negative pressure to the patient's body (and consequently to the chest wall) supported inspiration, creating a subatmospheric pressure, and expiration was a passive process. Over the years, NIV has continued to evolve. Although some NIV techniques that apply an alternate external negative pressure to the chest wall, such as the cuirass and poncho wrap, still exist, they have mostly been abandoned [1, 6]. Nowadays, the most common NIV modalities provide a positive pressure synchronized with the patient's inspiration.

NIV has become one of the most important tools in the hands of clinicians for dealing with acute respiratory failure (ARF) of different causes, especially exacerbation of chronic obstructive pulmonary disease (COPD) and acute cardiogenic edema [7, 8]. NIV can also be used as a continuous or intermittent ventilatory support in patients with chronic respiratory failure. COPD and obstructive sleep apnea syndrome (OSAS), as well as chest wall restrictive disease and neuromuscular disease, can benefit from NIV even in a domiciliary environment [1]. During the corona-virus disease 2019 (COVID-19) outbreak, NIV was shown to be a valid means of ventilatory support for many patients with ARF in an emergency scenario where the optimization of resources played a pivotal role. Non-invasive modes of ventilation were commonly used as a first-line tool in selected patients with COVID-19 pneumonia [5]. NIV can also be used for palliative purposes, providing respiratory support for patients who refuse intubation but still need supportive therapies, and in patients who need to alleviate terminal symptoms, especially dyspnea [9].

This chapter summarizes and clarifies why and when to start NIV in acute and chronic critically ill patients, focusing on each of the most common diseases in the intensive care unit (ICU) setting.

5.2 General Criteria for Starting NIV

5.2.1 Indications and Contraindications of NIV

Among the various causes of ARF, a few general criteria can be rapidly evaluated to identify a patient who could benefit from ventilatory support. It is highly recommended to start ventilatory support when the following signs and symptoms are present [1, 7, 10]: (1) signs of respiratory distress or dyspnea; (2) an increased respiratory rate compared with the patient's baseline rate; (3) activation of accessory respiratory muscles (i.e., scalene, sternocleidomastoid, pectoralis major, trapezius, and external intercostal); (4) blood gas analysis showing signs of respiratory failure (arterial oxygen tension/inspiratory oxygen fraction ratio $PaO_2/FIO_2 < 200$), hypercapnia with respiratory acidosis (arterial partial pressure of carbon dioxide, $PaCO_2 > 45$ mmHg and pHa $<$ 7.35), and/or hypoxemia ($PaO_2 < 60$ mmHg). In a situation when these criteria coexist, NIV can be initiated, but some exclusion criteria must be assessed before starting a non-invasive treatment; those criteria can be considered as absolute or relative contraindications [1, 9].

Absolute contraindications include (1) respiratory arrest; (2) coma and loss of upper protective airways reflexes; (3) severe hemodynamic instability (i.e., acute myocardial infarction, hemodynamic shock); (4) facial deformity that precludes the application of the interface (i.e., post-traumatic or post-surgery lesions and facial burns); (5) obstruction of upper airways; and (6) recent (<2 weeks) esophagectomy.

Relative contraindications include (1) drowsiness or Glasgow Coma Scale <8 points, cognitive impairment, or agitation; (2) vomiting or the presence of secretions in the upper airways with a risk of inhalation; (3) abdominal distension; (4) acute pneumothorax. Drowsiness and cognitive impairment could be symptoms of acute hypercapnia, and NIV should be considered to improve gas exchange [11, 12]. In the case of agitation, the use of a sedative agent such as dexmedetomidine is suggested to improve the tolerance to NIV treatment [7] and synchrony with the ventilator. In the case of vomiting, a nasogastric tube could be placed and maintained during NIV treatment. Acute pneumothorax should be promptly managed, although NIV could be considered to apply low positive pressure support in selected cases. When NIV is started in the presence of a relative contraindication, the patient should be under accurate supervision [13] in an appropriate hospital location.

5.2.2 Selection of Patients Who Can Benefit from NIV

An important step before starting NIV is evaluation of the patient's history to determine the possible cause of ARF, as well as detection of patients who could benefit and those for whom NIV is contraindicated. The evidence strongly supports NIV treatment in patients with COPD exacerbation with concomitant respiratory acidosis [10, 14] and in patients with acute cardiogenic edema [10, 15]. In immunocompromised patients with ARF of different causes, early NIV is considered [9].

On the other hand, in patients with de novo respiratory failure (without previous episodes), pneumonia, and severe acute respiratory distress syndrome (ARDS), the available guidelines do not strictly recommend the use of NIV. This choice is justified by the fact that in these diseases, improvement in gas exchange, decrease in the work of breathing and dyspnea, and avoidance of endotracheal intubation are not easily achievable [9, 13].

NIV can be used after surgery and after a thoracic trauma; in both situations, NIV helps reduce pain caused by breathing chest movements, avoiding dysventilation. Other applications of NIV include support in the post-extubation period to prevent extubation failure [9, 13].

Patients affected by neuromuscular disease often present with chronic respiratory failure, restrictive pulmonary disease, and obstructive pulmonary disease. In these cases, NIV is commonly used to treat these patients, even in a domiciliary setting [1, 13].

5.2.3 Selection of the NIV Interface

After proper patient selection, subsequent steps are the choice of the interface and the ventilator settings. The correct choice of interface is a key point for the success of NIV. The NIV interfaces currently available and most often used include a nasal mask, oronasal mask, full-face mask, helmet, and nasal pillows. A helmet but mostly a full-face mask is most commonly used in cases of ARF [13], but they are not the first choice in a chronic domiciliary setting where a nasal mask is the interface of choice [16].

The interface is fundamental to connect the ventilator tubing to the patient's airways, creating a semi-open ventilatory circuit; by definition, this circuit could have leaks between the interface and the skin or through the mouth in case of a nasal mask. The ideal characteristics of the correct NIV interface should include (1) a proper cover of the patient's airways based on the patient's pattern of breathing (e.g., an oro-nasal mask if the patient is breathing with the mouth open); (2) the mask should be comfortable for the patient and avoid contact with previous facial ulcers; (3) the mask must be of the right size for the patient to minimize air leaks; air leaks could have an impact on patient-ventilator synchrony, affecting the efficiency of NIV [17], because they interfere with the ventilator's trigger and cycle phase [18]; the NIV interface also affects dead space; it does not affect the outcome of treatment but ventilator settings need to be adjusted [18, 19]; (4) humidification and warming of the gases used to protect the endotracheal epithelium and limit airway resistance [20]; (5) a successful strategy to obtain the most comfort for the patient could be turnover of different interfaces [19].

5.2.4 Selection of the Most Appropriate NIV Modality

The selection of an appropriate modality of NIV should focus on the patient's needs and the availability of NIV interfaces and ventilators. This should account for disease characteristics (e.g., hypercapnia vs hypocapnia) and the goals of each NIV modality. Moreover, the ventilator settings are an important part of NIV treatment and clinicians should know how to manage the mechanical ventilators available in their wards. Pressure-targeted modes are mostly used during NIV; they deliver a preselected inspiration pressure. In pressure support ventilation, the inspiration pressure is delivered starting from an end-positive expiratory pressure (EPAP); in bilevel support, the inspiration pressure is the maximum pressure level reached in the airways at the end of inspiration (inspiratory positive airway pressure, IPAP) over an EPAP; the pressure support is the difference between IPAP and EPAP [13]. Pressure-targeted modes are more comfortable for the patient than volume-targeted modes because they gradually apply the pressure to the airways and are better at compensating for air leaks [9]. The amount of pressure support is a clinical decision made with consideration of the patient's underlying disease and respiratory performance, keeping in mind that the tidal volume should be set on predicted body weight and an adequate respiratory rate. The most commonly used triggering systems are of the flow type; when the patient starts inspiration, part of the background flow in the ventilator circuit (called bias flow), which is read at the beginning of the inspiration by the ventilator, is subtracted before pressure support is delivered. It is now clear why it is important to minimize leaks because they can be erroneously read as a patient's inspiration effort. The sensitivity of the triggering system should be set both to avoid auto-triggering (not too high) and to recognize the beginning of inspiration (not too low). The expiratory phase of respiration begins after the pressurized flow falls below a fixed percentage of the pick of flow; the passage to the expiratory phase is called flow cycling and is characterized by opening of the expiratory valve in the ventilator, allowing the patient to exhale. Even in these circumstances, leaks could affect the reduction of flow and interfere with synchrony. ICU ventilators, even with proper settings, are more subject to patient-ventilator asynchrony than specifically designed ventilators for NIV, which perform better in compensating for leaks [9].

To summarize, the success of NIV is greatly affected by accurate selection of patients and good knowledge of NIV interfaces, ventilators, and ventilator settings.

In the 2000s, the use of a novel less invasive device became widespread: the high flow nasal oxygen (HFNO). An HFNO delivers oxygen with some peculiarities; it uses high flow gases (up to 60 L/min), reducing the dead space with a positive effect on carbon dioxide washout and improving the work of breathing with a reduction in the respiratory rate [21–23]. Another effect of high flow is the generation of a positive end-expiratory pressure (PEEP), but this effect is partially reduced by the opening of the mouth during respiration; however, levels of 2–3 cmH_2O PEEP are obtained with 45 and 50–60 L/min flux in optimal conditions (mouth closed) [22, 23], and this contributes to alveolar recruitment [22]. HFNO performs better in guaranteeing a constant FiO_2 in comparison with conventional oxygen therapy (COT) and Venturi masks, thanks to an oxygen blender connected to the circuit [22] or the direct use of a mechanical ventilator with proper settings [21]. The HFNO circuit also includes an active heated humidifier with the delivery of warm and humidified gas into the airways, which maintains mucosal function [23] and prevents ulceration, epithelial damage, and adhesive mucus [21]. In the last few years, research and trials have investigated the role of HFNCO in supporting patients with respiratory impairment. Although HFNO has an emerging role in the treatment of hypoxemic respiratory failure, further investigation are needed [22, 24].

5.3 Clinical Indications for Starting NIV in the Acute Setting

5.3.1 Acute Exacerbation of COPD

COPD is a respiratory disease whereby the inflammatory response to toxins (most often smoke toxins) in the bronchi epithelium obstructs the expiration flow. Patients with COPD usually tolerate mild hypoxia and hypercapnia well. During a COPD exacerbation, fatigue of the respiratory muscles and diaphragm leads to inadequate alveolar ventilation, increasing the $PaCO_2$ and causing respiratory acidosis. In addition, hyperinflation contributes to insufficient muscular activity [9]. Before starting NIV treatment in patients with COPD, blood gas analysis should be performed together with clinical evaluation of the respiratory rate, paying attention when it is >23 breaths/min, and respiratory mechanics; a chest radiograph is suggested but should not delay the treatment [13].

NIV treatment is recommended when increased arterial CO_2 leads to respiratory acidosis (pH < 7.35 and $PaCO_2$ > 45 mmHg), despite adequate O_2 and optimal medical therapy [7, 9, 10, 13]. NIV treatment is superior to O_2 therapy alone in reducing the need for endotracheal intubation and hospital length of stay [8]. NIV is the first-line therapy even in patients considered for endotracheal intubation, although a trial of NIV should be performed only if they are not rapidly deteriorating [9]. Furthermore, NIV is not inferior to IMV [25]. Bilevel NIV is the most effective NIV strategy suggested in the literature. The ventilatory settings suggested by the British Thoracic Society/Intensive Care Society guidelines for patients with hypercapnic ARF include titration of NIV parameters within the first 10–30 min, starting from an EPAP of 3 cmH_2O and IPAP of 15 cmH_2O (using an inspiratory time from 0.8 s to 1.2 s) up to 20 cmH_2O if pH < 7.5, to achieve normalization of the respiratory rate and respiratory mechanics [13]. NIV has shown its efficacy in patients with severe (pH < 7.20) and mild (pH 7.30–7.35) respiratory acidosis by improving the gas exchange within the first hour of treatment; the most effective results are seen when the health care personnel are highly trained for NIV treatment [26]. The use of NIV is not suggested to prevent respiratory acidosis in patients with hypercapnia alone. In those patients, medical therapy and O_2 should be titrated to obtain oxygen saturation of 88–92% [27], heal gas exchange, and permit decompensation and recovery of respiratory muscles. NIV treatment should not be interrupted frequently. The discontinuation of NIV could be considered when pHa and $PaCO_2$ return to normal values together with improved patient condition.

Regarding the effects on outcome, NIV during COPD exacerbation has proven its efficacy in reducing the risk of mortality up to 46% and endotracheal intubation up to 64% in comparison with usual care. In addition, when NIV is associated with standard therapy, the hospital length of stay is reduced by up to 3 days [28]. These important results are sustained in the literature both in the ICU and general ward setting.

5.3.2 Acute Cardiogenic Pulmonary Edema

During acute cardiogenic pulmonary edema (ACPE), the accumulation of fluid in the lungs leads to impairment in gas exchange with a shunt effect (impairment between ventilation and perfusion in a lung area that fails to oxygenate the blood). The underlying mechanisms of this retention could be an increased left ventricular (LV) afterload and/or a left ventricular diastolic dysfunction or a valvular dysfunction [29], which increases the pulmonary capillary hydrostatic pressure. The edema is the result of increased filtration of water in the extra-lung tissue, which overcomes the capacity of lymphatic drainage [30], and its presence is responsible for minor lungs participating in gas exchange, increased airway resistance, and major work in breathing [19]. Diagnostic criteria for ACPE are dyspnea (which worsens in the orthostatic position, orthopnea), tachypnea (respiratory rate > 25 breaths/min), increased work of breathing, and ARF with hypoxemia and sometimes hypercapnia (peripheral saturation of oxygen, $SpO_2 < 90\%$ in room air, arterial blood gases $PaO_2 < 60$ mmHg, $PaCO_2 > 45$ mmHg) [10]. Two of the following findings are required to confirm ACPE: signs of pulmonary congestion on a chest radiograph or CT scan, lung ultrasonography showing B lines, increased pulmonary pressure on catheterization of the pulmonary artery with a Swan-Ganz catheter, increased total extravascular lung water identified with thermodilution techniques, presenting increased filling pressure and atrial natriuretic peptide [15].

Based on the above-mentioned physiologic mechanisms of the formation of ACPE, the reason for adopting NIV as a possible treatment both for cardiac and pulmonary purposes becomes clearer. The first step of ACPE treatment is based on oxygen delivery and medical therapy (diuretics to improve elimination of fluids and vasodilators to reduce systolic blood pressure and LV afterload). When ARF occurs ($SpO_2 < 90\%$ or $PaO_2 < 60$ mmHg), oxygen therapy is indicated and could be delivered both as a continuous positive airway pressure (CPAP) or NIV with pressure support (non-invasive mechanical ventilation [NIMV]) [9, 15, 29]. The reason why NIV and CPAP are recommended in ARF due to ACPE is because the application of positive intrathoracic pressure (PIP) limits the venous return and consequently the right ventricular preload, the LV preload, and systolic pressure; it also reduces the LV afterload by reducing the transmural ventricular pressure [1, 19]. PIP recruits the collapsed alveoli, improving shunt and gas exchange and applying pressure that reverses water filtration in the lungs [15]. The reason is that they both rapidly improve dyspnea, gas exchange, and the work of breathing with a significant decrease in mortality [17, 23] and need for endotracheal intubation in comparison with traditional oxygen therapy; currently, there is no evidence that one modality is preferred to the other [9, 15, 29]. NIV and CPAP also probably reduce the hospital length of stay in those patients [32], but this needs more trials because the literature does not agree on this outcome. The superiority of NIV over traditional oxygen therapy has been proven, even in the prehospital setting, to treat ACPE manifesting with $SpO_2 < 90\%$ and clinical signs of ARF, but it should not delay hospital admission; its use significantly reduces the intubation rate [31]. However, NIV in the prehospital setting needs further studies to improve the evidence.

ACPE can occur with acute heart failure due to acute cardiogenic shock or acute coronary syndrome. Those patients are usually excluded in trials that investigate the use of NIV in ACPE, so the previous recommendation is not suggested for this group of patients [9], even if there is probably no difference between NIV and standard medical treatment in the incidence of myocardial infarction [32].

5.3.3 Acute Exacerbation of Asthma

During acute exacerbation of asthma, ARF occurs consequent to sudden bronchoconstriction, which causes increased airway resistance with hyperinflation. Patients manifest dyspnea and increased work of breathing, which could worsen with patient's exhaustion due to hypercapnia.

Overall, the literature and recent guidelines [9, 13] do not recommend the use of NIV in addition to medical treatment or as first-line ventilatory support for ARF in this group of patients due to the lack of available strong randomized clinical trials (RCTs) that confirm the efficacy of NIV in reducing mortality, intubation rates, and ICU and hospital length of stay [9, 33, 34] and the low mortality rate in patients treated with IMV [13]. However, in the last few years, NIV has been tested in acute exacerbation of asthma. The increased confidence of clinicians in NIV and better selection of patients could be responsible for the reduction in failure of NIV [35] and its safe use [36], such as seen in some studies, but its reliability should be tested in an RCT [34, 37]. The Expert Panel Report 3 [38] (EPR-3) and updates [39] underline that accurate monitoring of signs and symptoms of worsening respiratory failure (deterioration in mental status, worsening hypercapnia, exhaustion) may indicate the need for prompt endotracheal intubation. Endotracheal intubation should not be delayed for an NIV trial, because it is a possible high-risk procedure due to the high risk of cardiocirculatory collapse on induction of anesthesia [40]. Therefore, we can conclude that in this group of patients, NIV should be cautiously considered, and further studies are warranted.

5.3.4 De Novo Acute Respiratory Failure

In de novo ARF, patients present to clinicians usually with significant hypoxemia (PaO_2/$FIO_2 \leq 300$) and high respiratory rate (>30–35 breaths/min), excluding certain causes of respiratory deterioration such as exacerbation of COPD, acute cardiogenic edema [1], previous pulmonary disease, and post-extubation and postoperative period [9]. The most frequent illnesses seen in these patients are pneumonia and ARDS.

The first purpose of NIV is to reduce the work of breathing, but in this group of patients, it is not easy to achieve. Therefore, recent guidelines [9] do not provide a recommendation for NIV in de novo ARF. The topic has been widely investigated in the literature and results are not univocal. A recent meta-analysis by Zayed et al. [41] compared NIV, HFNC, and COT in de novo ARF and showed a reduction in the intubation rate in the NIV group in comparison with COT, but no difference was seen in the reduction of short- and long-term mortality. Comparing NIV with HFNC and HFNC with COT, there was no significant difference among the different treatments in reduction of intubation rate and mortality. Frat et al. [42] investigated the potential benefits of HFNC, NIV, and COT in patients with ARF with-

out hypercapnia; there was no difference in reduction of the intubation rate, but there was a significantly higher performance of HFNC in reduction of 90-day mortality. Lee et al. [43] reported that HFNC may be superior to COT, but its superiority in terms of a reduction in mortality needs to be tested in further clinical trials.

NIV could reduce the inspiration effort in patients with ARDS compared with no ventilatory assistance, but the application of sufficient pressure support could lead to high tidal volumes and transpulmonary pressure, which are undesirable in the lung-protective approach that is usually recommended [9, 13]. Some new evidence suggests that patients with ARDS and mild oxygen impairment (PaO_2/$FiO_2 > 200$ mmHg) could benefit from spontaneous breathing and non-invasive strategies in terms of reduction in the intubation rate [44]. Patients with moderate or severe ARDS (with a PaO_2/$FiO_2 < 200$) are a more delicate population where the balance between the potential harm of spontaneous breathing and the known benefit of NIV is still debated; among these patients, HFNC and helmet NIV could be new tools, but their efficiency needs to be established [4, 44–46]. The effectiveness and safety of NIV are constantly being investigated; in a single-center RCT, helmet NIV has been shown to reduce the need for endotracheal intubation and improve the long-term survival in comparison to face mask NIV [47]. What is certain is that every non-invasive approach should be applied under strict surveillance because a delay in starting IMV leads to bad outcomes [9].

5.3.5 Coronavirus Disease-2019

Patients with COVID-19 could manifest a wide range of symptom severity; they could be completely asymptomatic or be affected by life-threatening ARF [48, 49]. Because of the complex pathophysiology that underlies COVID-19 disease, which has some similarities with ARDS, the clinical approach should be personalized based on the clinical findings [50]. Oxygen therapy in a patient with COVID-19 aims to improve

ARF, and NIV has been used since the beginning of pandemic even though there was, and still is, uncertainty regarding its effects on outcome [51, 52]. The Surviving Sepsis Campaign (SSC) Guidelines for the Management of Critically Ill Adults with COVID-19 [53] suggest using oxygen therapy when the SpO_2 is <92% and recommend oxygen therapy when SpO_2 is <90%. Despite its widespread availability and simplicity in use, COT cannot provide respiratory support and is not recommended in patients with ARF due to COVID-19 [5, 53]. HFNO is suggested over COT [53]; HFNO may reduce the risk of endotracheal intubation [54], but it is not associated with a reduction in mortality or ICU length of stay [55, 56]. On the other hand, CPAP delivered with a helmet showed a success rate of 60% in patients with COVID-19 [57], whereas in the HENIVOT trial, helmet NIV showed no difference in reducing the intubation rate using HFNO, but interestingly it seemed to improve the days free of respiratory support [58]. Due to the variability of the results, more RCTs should be performed to assess the impact of NIV in patients with COVID-19 [51]. The SSC guidelines suggest the use of HFNO when available over NIV; in the absence of HFNO, an NIV trial (either with a helmet or face mask) could be performed under close surveillance and if there is no evidence of the need for intubation [53]. Endotracheal intubation should not be delayed [59] and should be performed preferentially within 3–8 h of the respiratory rate > 28 breaths/min and/or PaO_2/FiO_2 that does not improve and/or $PaCO_2$ < 30 mmHg [60].

5.3.6 Weaning from Invasive Mechanical Ventilation

Recent guidelines [9, 13] suggest the use of NIV when weaning patients with hypercapnic respiratory failure from IMV, especially those with COPD exacerbation. In this population, compared with classic weaning protocols based on reduction of pressure support or spontaneous breathing trials (SBTs), NIV reduces weaning failure, ventilator-associated pneumonia, ICU and hospital length of stay, and duration of mechanical ventilation and invasive mechanical ventilation. In hypoxemic ARF, the same guidelines do not support the use of NIV due to the lack of proof of efficiency. In a recent meta-analysis, Shan et al. [61] concluded that weaning using NIV methods, instead of invasive weaning, did not decrease hospital mortality, but reduced ICU length of stay and adverse events. However, large RCTs are needed to provide stronger evidence.

5.3.7 NIV in the Prevention and Treatment of ARF after Extubation

Successful extubation occurs when a patient does not need ventilatory support in the following 48 h [13]. General risk factors for weaning failure are presented in the Table 5.1 [13]. NIV support has been tested for the prevention of ARF after extubation. According to the literature, patients are separated into two major groups: unselected patients and at-risk patients. The different pathophysiology of hypercapnic and normocapnic ARF can explain the different results of weaning trials; atelectasis, accumulation of bronchial secretion, and hypoventilation are most frequent

Table 5.1 Risk factors for NIV failure

Hemodynamic	Positive fluid balance
	Hemodynamic instability
Respiratory	Previous failed extubation
	Increased rapid shallow breathing index during spontaneous breathing trial
	Pneumonia or pulmonary disease as the cause requiring IMV
	Prolonged duration of IMV
Neurologic	Loss of consciousness (i.e., bulbar dysfunction)
	Delirium, agitation
Patient factors	Low albumin
	Increased age
	Anemia
	Increased severity of illness

IMV invasive mechanical ventilation, *NIV* non-invasive ventilation factors responsible for hypoxemic ARF, but they are not improved by NIV. NIV was found to prevent ARF in the post-extubation period only in the at-risk group [9, 13]; patients in this group are usually older than 65 years and have an underlying respiratory or cardiac disease. In those patients, affected by a re-intubation risk of 20–30%, NIV decreases this risk together with the risk of mortality. Patients without risk factors should not receive NIV to prevent ARF after extubation because it does not change the re-intubation rate or mortality [9]. When ARF is established in the early post-extubation period, NIV should not be used. More evidence is needed in this scenario, but the available data suggest that the use of NIV could have negative effects on patient outcomes, such as increased mortality, probably due to the delay in re-intubation [9, 13]. An NIV trial could be justified only in patients with COPD in the hands of expert clinicians [13].

5.3.8 NIV in Palliative Care

In a palliative care setting, patients and their families expect alleviation of symptoms more than resolution of the clinical status. Based on findings of the Society of Critical Care Medicine Task Force [62] and a few other RCTs, the European Respiratory Society (ERS)/American Thoracic Society (ATS) guidelines [9] suggest NIV for dyspneic patients with terminal conditions. Patients' preferences must be established to know how far support therapy should be applied, and NIV could also be applied to give the patient time to understand their desires [13]. In patients for whom the goal is not survival but reduction of terminal symptoms for the last hours of life, NIV could improve breathlessness and respiratory distress without a negative impact on cognition and communication, which can be experienced with the use of opioids. In patients who forego intubation but the goal is to survive hospitalization, NIV is not recommended in the guidelines [9] for lack of evidence, but it seems to improve hospital survival in patients with COPD and congestive heart failure in some RCTs. Death during NIV support could be comfortable and

removal is not necessary, but a healthcare professional should be trained to give the best palliative support [13].

5.4 NIV in the Chronic Setting

5.4.1 Long-Term NIV in COPD

Recently, the ERS and the ATS published some recommendations for an evidence-based approach to COPD. COPD could induce stable chronic respiratory failure (CRF) with hypercapnia and/or hypoxemia [63] worsening the patient's quality of life (QoL). Lungs are hyperinflated as a consequence of incremented airway resistance due to emphysema and alternated small lower airways. Hyperinflation and pathologic muscular atrophy have a negative impact on the efficiency of the diaphragm with increased work of breathing and hypercapnia [64]. In those patients, hypercapnia is defined as FEV_1/forced vital capacity (FVC) <0.70 plus $PaCO_2$ > 45 mmHg at rest (not during exacerbation). Long-term NIV could improve the respiratory parameters and gas exchange, symptoms (dyspnea, functional capacity), sleep, and QoL [65] by supporting muscular dysfunction and diaphragmatic insufficiency [64]. Both guidelines suggest the use of long-term NIV, which seems to have a positive impact on chronic COPD symptoms, especially dyspnea but also exercise tolerance and QoL; less impact was seen on the improvement of sleep quality. Even if starting long-term NIV treatment means facing the cost of administration and monitoring, which could be a limitation to the widespread use of domiciliary NIV in some cases, it seems to have a positive impact on the burden of hospital admission and exacerbation of COPD. The ERS guidelines suggest the use of long-term NIV after severe hypercapnic ARF if hypercapnia persists after the resolution of exacerbation because of the potential reduction of exacerbation and hospitalizations. Guidelines give a conditional recommendation because patients could continue to improve in the 2–4 weeks after discharge (based on the results of the RCTs [63]), and they should be evaluated again to test the need for long-term NIV. On this topic, the ATS guidelines do not suggest the use of NIV in hypercapnic patients with COPD; the expert panel underlines that the results of the HOT-HMV trial showed that not all patients were hypercapnic 2–4 weeks after the initial episode, so the application of long-term NIV may eventually be not necessary. In addition, starting long-term NIV in the hospital setting could benefit from the support from starting treatment in the hands of experts, but prolong hospitalizations and costs. The ATS guidelines also suggest screening patients for obstructive sleep apnea (OSA) before the initiation of treatment; in patients with a COPD-OSA overlap, OSA and obesity could be important contributors to hypoventilation more than COPD. Assessing the coexistence of those diseases could lead to better management of home mechanical ventilation when choosing CPAP or NIV, levels of EPAP, and use or discontinuation of inhalers.

Interesting results were reported in the RCT of Duiverman et al. [66] who compared starting NIV treatment at home (monitored by telemedicine) and in-hospital NIV initiation in stable hypercapnic patients with COPD. In this study, home initiation of treatment was not inferior in improving daytime $PaCO_2$, QoL, and exercise tolerance. In addition, pulmonary rehabilitation improved the compliance and efficiency of domiciliary NIV treatment.

5.4.2 Obstructive Sleep Apnea Syndrome and Obesity Hypoventilation Syndrome

In OSAS, the partial or total collapse of upper airways leads to bad quality of sleep with arousals and desaturation. Causes are different but manifestations are similar: decreased cognitive performance, fatigue, headache, sleepiness during the day, and snoring and choking during sleep [67, 68]. Obesity is common in these patients and seems to contribute to a loss of muscular tone with a reduction in the oropharyngeal space, mainly at the end of exhalation, contributing to increased work of breathing. Strong evidence supports the use of CPAP in OSAS; it can improve daytime cognitive function and wakefulness, quality of sleep, and overall QoL [68].

Obesity hypoventilation syndrome (OHS) causes daytime hypercapnia and CRF with no evident cause of hypoventilation apart from increased body mass index (BMI). Progressive retention of CO_2 caused by repetitive obstruction of airways could be responsible for daytime hypercapnia [69]. Patients with OSAS have OHS in 20–30% of cases [68] (especially when BMI >40 kg/m^2) and 73% of patients with OHS have concomitant OSAS [70], so there is an important overlap of the two syndromes. In patients with a pure form of OHS with little contribution of OSAS, CPAP has a limited effect because hypoventilation is the most important factor, more than obstruction. Bilevel NIV could treat the hypoventilation seen in pure OHS. Two different studies of Masa et al. [69, 70] tested NIV on patients with OHS. Bilevel NIV improved $PaCO_2$, serum bicarbonate, polysomnographic apnea-hypopnea index (AHI, an index of severity of sleep apnea; it represents the number of apnea and hypopnea for an hour of sleep) and nocturnal oxygenation independently of NIV compliance in the cohort of patients with OHS without OSAS. In the Pickwick study [70], patients with OHS and OSAS treated with NIV and CPAP showed improvement in nocturnal oxygenation and sleep quality in comparison with the control group treated with lifestyle modification only. In the comparison between the control group, CPAP and NIV, the latter demonstrated superior results in the improvement in $PaCO_2$ and serum bicarbonate. Indications for NIV in patients with OSAS and those with hypoventilation syndrome [68] are shown in Fig. 5.1.

5.4.3 NIV in Thoracic Restrictive Disorders and Neuromuscular Disease

Thoracic restrictive disorders (TRD) and neuromuscular disease (NMD) could be characterized by CRF. In TRD, the respiratory drive is intact, but the abnormalities of the thoracic cage are responsible for inadequate ventilation and

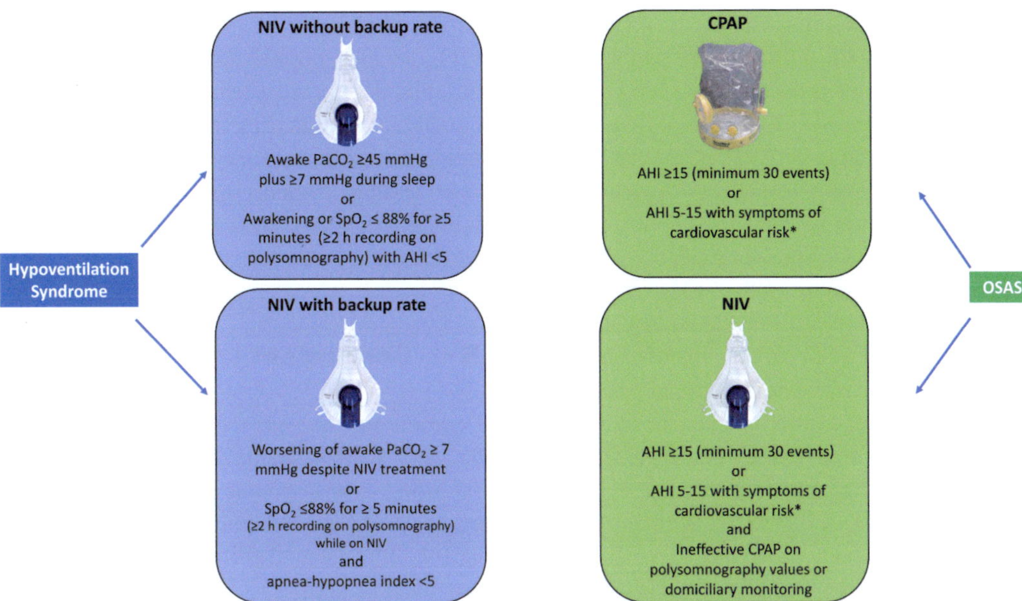

Fig. 5.1 Indications for NIV in patients with obstructive sleep apnea syndrome and hypoventilation syndrome. *Significant daytime sleepiness, altered cognition, mood disorders, insomnia, hypertension, ischemic heart disease, previous stroke. *AHI* apnea-hypopnea index, *CPAP* con-tinuous positive airway pressure, *NIV* non-invasive venti-lation, *OSAS* obstructive sleep apnea syndrome, *PaCO₂* arterial partial pressure of carbon dioxide, *SpO₂* peripheral saturation of oxygen

increased work of breathing, which results in hypercapnia; the most common diseases with these characteristics are scoliosis and kyphosis, and thoracoplasty could also lead to these conse-quences. Hypercapnia may be detected first dur-ing rapid eye movement sleep before its presentation in later phases of the disease, during nonrapid eye movement (NREM) sleep and wakefulness [71].

In NMD, progressive muscular dysfunction affects even respiratory muscles with a reduction in strength, progressive reduction of alveolar ventilation, and impairment in clearance of secre-tions. Hypoventilation can lead to hypoxemia and hypercapnia, but dyspnea is a late symptom because these patients usually do not move and do not need to increase their vital capacity (VC) during muscular effort; respiratory function fol-low-up with spirometry can be used for monitor-ing lung function and anticipate nocturnal hypercapnia; VC <680 mL is sensitive for day-time hypercapnia. NMD can be classified as rap-idly progressive with worsening of muscular

function over months, as in amyotrophic lateral sclerosis (ALS), and relatively rapid progressive in which muscular function worsens over a few years, as in Duchenne muscular dystrophy (DMD); life expectancy is reduced overall [72].

The goals of NIV treatment in these patients are to put respiratory muscle at rest, reestablish the correct CO_2 sensitivity of the central ventila-tion control neurons, and support pulmonary mechanics [73].

Indications for NIV treatment in patients with TRD [1] include (1) symptoms of hypoventila-tion; and (2) at least one of the following signs: daytime $PaCO_2$ > 45 mmHg, $PaCO_2$ > 50 mmHg during sleep, daytime normocapnia worsening during sleep to <10 mmHg on percutaneous oximetry. Patients with RTD should be strictly monitored when they do not manifest daytime hypercapnia, but they have a VC of less than 50% of predicted values.

Indications for NIV treatment in patients with NMD [1, 68, 74] include (1) symptoms of hypoventilation; and (2) at least one of the following signs: daytime $PaCO_2$ > 45 mmHg, $PaCO_2$ > 45 mmHg during sleep, percutaneous oximetry >50 mmHg during sleep for >30 min; and (3) in patients with ALS or rapidly progressive NMD, reduction of FVC >10% from baseline. In this subgroup, respiratory symptoms are mandatory for starting NIV treatment when the maximum inspiratory pressure is ≤60 mmHg or sniff nasal pressure is <40 mmHg or FVC is ≤50% of predicted. NIV in patients with ALS should be started when patients manifest oropharyngeal muscles weakness, bulbar symptoms with sialorrhea or aspiration risk, or inefficient cough [1]. In a systematic review by Hannan et al. [75], the impact of NIV treatment was greatest for TRD with improvement in the following parameters: dyspnea, somnolence, fatigue, and physical and mental health. This group of patients usually has more stable disease than those with NMD, and this could be the reason for better outcomes. In patients with ALS, NIV improved somnolence, fatigue, QoL, and prolonged survival (survival rate was not improved in patients with major bulbar involvement). NIV improved survival even in patients with DMD with hypercapnic respiratory failure; patients with nocturnal hypoventilation are at risk of daytime hypercapnia and could benefit from early initiation of NIV. The REINVENT international survey by Periucci et al. [76] summarized the most important reasons to start NIV: diurnal hypercapnia, hospitalization for ARF, symptoms of muscular weakness, and nocturnal hypercapnia. This survey highlights that the major goal with NIV treatment was improvement in QoL and quality of sleep more than survival. Treatment compliance and patient feedback received high importance. The most common mode of ventilation used for day and night treatment was spontaneous timed pressure support ventilation and the most comfortable interface chosen for daytime NIV was a mouthpiece; oronasal masks were preferred overnight. The Dutch Homerun Trial [77] supports the beginning of NIV in TRD and NMD in a domiciliary setting; results of the RCT highlight that initiation of NIV at home was not inferior to in-hospital initiation in terms of improved daytime $PaCO_2$, nocturnal transcutaneous CO_2 exchange, PaO_2, and serum bicarbonate level. The results from QoL questionnaires and compliance during treatment were not different in the two groups. These findings support the initiation of NIV treatment in an out-of-hospital and more familiar environment.

5.5 Conclusions

NIV techniques are subject to continuous discussion and improvement. Although they have established strong support in certain conditions, such as COPD exacerbation or ACPE, their role is still highly debated for other conditions, and more clinical trials are needed to understand their efficacy and limits. What is certain is that well-trained staff is key to the success of treatment; the clinician's ability to use different modes of NIV and interfaces opens up a wide range of possibilities to give support to patients with impaired respiratory function to avoid invasive mechanical ventilation and its potential complications.

References

1. Torri G, Calderini E. Ventilazione artificiale meccanica - I supporti agli scambi respiratori. 3rd ed. Antonio Delfino Editore; 2020.
2. Brochard L. Mechanical ventilation: invasive versus noninvasive. Eur Respir J. 2003;22:31s–7s.
3. Tobin MJ. Principles and practice of mechanical ventilation. 3rd ed. McGraw-Hill; 2012.
4. Grieco DL, Menga LS, Eleuteri D, Antonelli M. Patient self-inflicted lung injury: implications for acute hypoxemic respiratory failure and ARDS patients on non-invasive support. Minerva Anestesiol. 2019;85:1014–23.
5. Battaglini D, et al. Noninvasive respiratory support and patient self-inflicted lung injury in COVID-19: a narrative review. Br J Anaesth. 2021;127:353–64.
6. Corrado A, Gorini M. Negative-pressure ventilation: is there still a role? Eur Respir J. 2002;20:187–97.
7. Hess DR. Noninvasive ventilation for acute respiratory failure. Respir Care. 2013;58:950–72.
8. Mas A, Masip J. Noninvasive ventilation in acute respiratory failure. COPD. 2014;9:837–52.

9. Rochwerg B, et al. Official ERS/ATS clinical practice guidelines: noninvasive ventilation for acute respiratory failure. Eur Respir J. 2017;50:1602426.

10. Ghosh D, Elliott MW. Acute non-invasive ventilation – getting it right on the acute medical take. Clin Med (Lond). 2019;19:237–42.

11. Scala R, Naldi M, Archinucci I, Coniglio G, Nava S. Noninvasive positive pressure ventilation in patients with acute exacerbations of COPD and varying levels of consciousness. Chest. 2005;128:1657–66.

12. Díaz GG, et al. Noninvasive positive-pressure ventilation to treat hypercapnic coma secondary to respiratory failure. Chest. 2005;127:952–60.

13. Davidson AC, et al. BTS/ICS guideline for the ventilatory management of acute hypercapnic respiratory failure in adults. Thorax. 2016;71(Suppl 2):ii1–35.

14. Ozsancak Ugurlu A, Habesoglu MA. Epidemiology of NIV for acute respiratory failure in COPD patients: results from the international surveys vs. the 'real world'. COPD. 2017;14:429–38.

15. Masip J, et al. Indications and practical approach to non-invasive ventilation in acute heart failure. Eur Heart J. 2018;39:17–25.

16. Storre JH, et al. Home noninvasive ventilatory support for patients with chronic obstructive pulmonary disease: patient selection and perspectives. Int J Chron Obstruct Pulmon Dis. 2018;13:753–60.

17. Otair HAA, BaHammam AS. Ventilator- and interface-related factors influencing patient-ventilator asynchrony during noninvasive ventilation. Ann Thorac Med. 2020;15:1.

18. Pisani L, Carlucci A, Nava S. Interfaces for noninvasive mechanical ventilation: technical aspects and efficiency. Minerva Anestesiol. 2012;78:1154–61.

19. Bello G, De Pascale G, Antonelli M. Noninvasive ventilation: practical advice. Curr Opin Crit Care. 2013;19:1–8.

20. Tuggey JM, Delmastro M, Elliott MW. The effect of mouth leak and humidification during nasal non-invasive ventilation. Respir Med. 2007;101:1874–9.

21. Nishimura M. High-flow nasal cannula oxygen therapy devices. Respir Care. 2019;64:735–42.

22. Mg D. High-flow nasal cannula oxygen in adults: an evidence-based assessment. Ann Am Thorac Soc. 2018;15:145–55.

23. Spicuzza L, Schisano M. High-flow nasal cannula oxygen therapy as an emerging option for respiratory failure: the present and the future. Ther Adv Chronic Dis. 2020;11:2040622320920106.

24. Rochwerg B, et al. The role for high flow nasal cannula as a respiratory support strategy in adults: a clinical practice guideline. Intensive Care Med. 2020;46:2226–37.

25. Conti G, et al. Noninvasive vs. conventional mechanical ventilation in patients with chronic obstructive pulmonary disease after failure of medical treatment in the ward: a randomized trial. Intensive Care Med. 2002;28:1701–7.

26. Comellini V, Pacilli AMG, Nava S. Benefits of non-invasive ventilation in acute hypercapnic respiratory failure. Respirology. 2019;24:308–17.

27. O'Driscoll BR, Howard LS, Davison AG. BTS guideline for emergency oxygen use in adult patients. Thorax. 2008;63:vi1–vi68.

28. Osadnik CR, et al. Non-invasive ventilation for the management of acute hypercapnic respiratory failure due to exacerbation of chronic obstructive pulmonary disease. Cochrane Database Syst Rev. 2017;7:CD004104.

29. ESC Scientific Document Group. 2021 ESC Guidelines for the diagnosis and treatment of acute and chronic heart failure. Eur Heart J. 2021;42(36):3599–726. https://www.escardio.org/Guidelines/Clinical-Practice-Guidelines/Acute-and-Chronic-Heart-Failure

30. Ware LB, Matthay MA. Acute pulmonary edema. N Engl J Med. 2005;353:2788–96.

31. Abubacker AP, et al. Non-invasive positive pressure ventilation for acute cardiogenic pulmonary edema and chronic obstructive pulmonary disease in prehospital and emergency settings. Cureus. 2021;13:e15624.

32. Berbenetz N, et al. Non-invasive positive pressure ventilation (CPAP or bilevel NPPV) for cardiogenic pulmonary oedema. Cochrane Database Syst Rev. 2019;4:CD005351.

33. Fergeson JE, Patel SS, Lockey RF. Acute asthma, prognosis, and treatment. J Allergy Clin Immunol. 2017;139:438–47.

34. Lim WJ, et al. Non-invasive positive pressure ventilation for treatment of respiratory failure due to severe acute exacerbations of asthma. Cochrane Database Syst Rev. 2012;12:CD004360.

35. Manglani R, et al. The use of non- invasive ventilation in asthma exacerbation - a two year retrospective analysis of outcomes. J Community Hosp Intern Med Perspect. 2021;11:727–32.

36. Miller A, VanHart DA, Gentile MA. Noninvasive ventilation in life-threatening asthma: a case series. Can J Respir Ther. 2017;53:33–6.

37. Landry A, Foran M, Koyfman A. Does noninvasive positive-pressure ventilation improve outcomes in severe asthma exacerbations? Ann Emerg Med. 2013;62:594–6.

38. National Asthma Education and Prevention Program, Third expert panel on the diagnosis and management of asthma. Expert panel report 3: guidelines for the diagnosis and management of asthma. National Heart, Lung, and Blood Institute (US) 2007.

39. National Heart, Lung, and Blood Institute. asthma management guidelines: focused updates 2020. NHLBI, NIH 2020. https://www.nhlbi.nih.gov/health-topics/asthma-management-guidelines-2020-updates.

40. D'Amato G, et al. Near fatal asthma: treatment and prevention. Eur Ann Allergy Clin Immunol. 2016;48:116–22.

41. Zayed Y, et al. Initial noninvasive oxygenation strategies in subjects with de novo acute hypoxemic respiratory failure. Respir Care. 2019;64:1433–44.

42. Frat J-P, et al. High-flow oxygen through nasal cannula in acute hypoxemic respiratory failure. N Engl J Med. 2015;372:2185–96.

43. Lee CC, et al. High flow nasal cannula versus conventional oxygen therapy and non-invasive ventilation in adults with acute hypoxemic respiratory failure: a systematic review. Respir Med. 2016;121:100–8.

44. Grieco DL, et al. Non-invasive ventilatory support and high-flow nasal oxygen as first-line treatment of acute hypoxemic respiratory failure and ARDS. Intensive Care Med. 2021;47:851–66.

45. De Jong A, Hernandez G, Chiumello D. Is there still a place for noninvasive ventilation in acute hypoxemic respiratory failure? Intensive Care Med. 2018;44:2248–50.

46. Antonelli M. NIV through the helmet can be used as first-line intervention for early mild and moderate ARDS: an unproven idea thinking out of the box. Crit Care. 2019;23:146.

47. Patel BK, Wolfe KS, Pohlman AS, Hall JB, Kress JP. Effect of noninvasive ventilation delivered by helmet vs face mask on the rate of endotracheal intubation in patients with acute respiratory distress syndrome: a randomized clinical trial. JAMA. 2016;315:2435–41.

48. Huang C, et al. Clinical features of patients infected with 2019 novel coronavirus in Wuhan, China. Lancet. 2020;395:497–506.

49. Berlin DA, Gulick RM, Martinez FJ. Severe Covid-19. N Engl J Med. 2020;383:2451–60.

50. Robba C, Battaglini D, Pelosi P, Rocco PRM. Multiple organ dysfunction in SARS-CoV-2: MODS-CoV-2. Expert Rev Respir Med. 2020;14:865–8.

51. Wang Z, et al. The use of non-invasive ventilation in COVID-19: a systematic review. Int J Infect Dis. 2021;106:254–61.

52. Sivaloganathan AA, et al. Noninvasive ventilation for COVID-19-associated acute hypoxaemic respiratory failure: experience from a single centre. Br J Anaesth. 2020;125:e368–71.

53. Alhazzani W, et al. Surviving sepsis campaign: guidelines on the management of critically ill adults with coronavirus disease 2019 (COVID-19). Crit Care Med. 2020;48:e440–69.

54. Agarwal A, et al. High-flow nasal cannula for acute hypoxemic respiratory failure in patients with COVID-19: systematic reviews of effectiveness and its risks of aerosolization, dispersion, and infection transmission. Can J Anaesth. 2020;67:1217–48.

55. Demoule A, et al. High-flow nasal cannula in critically iii patients with severe COVID-19. Am J Respir Crit Care Med. 2020;202:1039–42.

56. Bonnet N, et al. High flow nasal oxygen therapy to avoid invasive mechanical ventilation in SARS-CoV-2 pneumonia: a retrospective study. Ann Intensive Care. 2021;11:37.

57. Bellani G, et al. Noninvasive ventilatory support of patients with COVID-19 outside the intensive care units (WARd-COVID). Ann Am Thorac Soc. 2021;18:1020–6.

58. Grieco DL, et al. Effect of helmet noninvasive ventilation vs high-flow nasal oxygen on days free of respiratory support in patients with COVID-19 and moderate to severe hypoxemic respiratory failure: the HENIVOT randomized clinical trial. JAMA. 2021;325:1731–43.

59. Ball L, et al. Early versus late intubation in COVID-19 patients failing helmet CPAP: a quantitative computed tomography study. Respir Physiol Neurobiol. 2022;301:103889.

60. Robba C, et al. Ten things you need to know about intensive care unit management of mechanically ventilated patients with COVID-19. Expert Rev Respir Med. 2021;15:1293–302.

61. Shan M, et al. Noninvasive ventilation as a weaning strategy in subjects with acute hypoxemic respiratory failure. Respir Care. 2020;65:1574–84.

62. Curtis JR, et al. Noninvasive positive pressure ventilation in critical and palliative care settings: understanding the goals of therapy. Crit Care Med. 2007;35:932–9.

63. Ergan B, et al. European respiratory society guidelines on long-term home non-invasive ventilation for management of COPD. Eur Respir J. 2019;54:1901003.

64. Coleman JM, Wolfe LF, Kalhan R. Noninvasive ventilation in chronic obstructive pulmonary disease. Ann Am Thorac Soc. 2019;16:1091–8.

65. Macrea M, et al. Long-term noninvasive ventilation in chronic stable hypercapnic chronic obstructive pulmonary disease. An official American thoracic society clinical practice guideline. Am J Respir Crit Care Med. 2020;202:e74–87.

66. Duiverman ML, et al. Home initiation of chronic non-invasive ventilation in COPD patients with chronic hypercapnic respiratory failure: a randomised controlled trial. Thorax. 2020;75:244–52.

67. Maspero C, Giannini L, Galbiati G, Rosso G, Farronato G. Obstructive sleep apnea syndrome: a literature review. Minerva Stomatol. 2015;64:97–109.

68. Nicolini A, et al. Non-invasive ventilation in the treatment of sleep-related breathing disorders: a review and update. Rev Port Pneumol. 2014;20:324–35.

69. Masa JF, et al. Non-invasive ventilation in obesity hypoventilation syndrome without severe obstructive sleep apnoea. Thorax. 2016;71:899–906.

70. Nasa JF, et al. Efficacy of different treatment alternatives for obesity hypoventilation syndrome. Pickwick study. Am J Respir Crit Care Med. 2015;192:86–95.

71. Shneerson JM, Simonds AK. Noninvasive ventilation for chest wall and neuromuscular disorders. Eur Respir J. 2002;20:480–7.

72. Ambrosino N, Carpenè N, Gherardi M. Chronic respiratory care for neuromuscular diseases in adults. Eur Respir J. 2009;34:444–51.

73. Clinical indications for noninvasive positive pressure ventilation in chronic respiratory failure due to restrictive lung disease, COPD, and nocturnal

hypoventilation--a consensus conference report. Chest. 1999;116:521–34.

74. The EFNS Task Force on Diagnosis and Management of Amyotrophic Lateral Sclerosis, et al. EFNS guidelines on the clinical management of amyotrophic lateral sclerosis (MALS) – revised report of an EFNS task force. Eur J Neurol. 2012;19:360–75.

75. Hannan LM, Dominelli GS, Chen Y-W, Darlene Reid W, Road J. Systematic review of non-invasive positive pressure ventilation for chronic respiratory failure. Respir Med. 2014;108:229–43.

76. Pierucci P, et al. REINVENT: ERS international survey on REstrictive thoracic diseases IN long term home noninvasive VENTilation. ERJ Open Res. 2021;7:00911–2020. https://doi.org/10.1183/23120541.00911-2020.

77. van den Biggelaar RJM, et al. A randomized trial of initiation of chronic noninvasive mechanical ventilation at home vs in-hospital in patients with neuromuscular disease and thoracic cage disorder: the dutch homerun trial. Chest. 2020;158:2493–501.

Critical Care Applications of NIMV and Related Issues: Pre-hospital and Emergency Medicine

Non-invasive Mechanical Ventilation in Prehospital Medicine

6

E. Taddei, G. Giuliano, D. Vannini, V. Motroni,
A. Cardu, A. Isirdi, C. Brusasco, F. Forfori,
and F. Corradi

Contents

E. Taddei (✉) · G. Giuliano · D. Vannini · V. Motroni
A. Cardu · A. Isirdi · C. Brusasco · F. Forfori
F. Corradi
Department of Surgical, Medical, Molecular
Pathology and Critical Care Medicine, University of
Pisa, Pisa, Italy
e-mail: claudia.brusasco@galliera.it;
francesco.forfori@unipi.it; francesco.corradi@unipi.it

6.1 Introduction

Dyspnea is defined by American Thoracic Society (ATS) as "a subjective experience of breathing discomfort that consists of qualitatively distinct sensations that vary in intensity" [1]. There are many causes of dyspnea that can be grouped into two main categories, i.e., lung failure and pump failure, in order to link the most appropriate treatment to pathophysiological mechanisms.

Dyspnea is a main cause of access to the emergency departments (ED), representing about 50% of all accesses in the USA and a frequent cause of activation of prehospital emergency services (10–50%) [2, 3]. Moreover, patients with dyspnea frequently develop respiratory failure requiring hospitalization (30–50%), intensive care (5–15%), with in-hospital mortality ranging from 5–10%, and ED mortality of 0.6% [2–4].

Acute respiratory failure (ARF) occurs when diseases of the heart or lungs lead to inadequate blood oxygen levels (hypoxia) or increased blood carbon dioxide levels (hypercapnia), eventually causing increased work of breathing and respiratory muscles fatigue [5].

As said above, the two categories of ARF involve several different etiologies and two large studies conducted in Europe and Asia (regarding access at ED) and Australia (more specific on prehospital setting) tried to stratify the main causes. These were the following: lower respiratory tract infections (14–30%), heart failure (15–20%), COPD exacerbation (13–18%), asthma (6–13%), acute myocardial infarction (3%), pulmonary embolism (2%), and other causes 33% (neuropathies, trauma, etc.) [2, 3].

In a study conducted by the National Institute for Healt Research [4], about 10% of patients developing ARF in prehospital settings reached the hospital with oxygen saturation (SpO_2) < 92%, despite standard oxygen therapy and mortality increased linearly with the distance to the definitive care structure (10% at 10 km, 20% at 20 km). This was possibly because treatments for acute hypoxaemic respiratory failure, particularly those involving respiratory support, are not readily available in prehospital settings. In addition, the definite treatment of ARF depends on the underlying cause, but this is difficult to be accurately determined in the ambulance while en route to hospital [6]. Thus, prehospital treatment of ARF often follows a common pathway [7], driven by clinical diagnostic criteria. For example, a clinical history of COPD or chronic heart failure (CHF), pharmacologic treatments, and auscultatory findings suggestive of CPE are taken for indication of NIV. Treatment options for patients with suspected asthma or COPD include nebulized salbutamol and ipratropium bromide, intramuscular adrenaline, and intravenous steroids.

Severe ARF in prehospital settings can be managed by invasively endotracheal intubation, which may be associated with complications, such as oral lacerations, aspiration, tube malposition, barotrauma, and VAP; the poorly controlled environment of prehospital settings increases the likelihood of these complications. Alternatively, ARF can be treated with NIV, which involves delivering oxygen under increased pressure via tight-fitting face mask, or helmet, or nasal cannulas [8].

NIV has been described as a "rational art" rather than application of science. It requires the ability of clinicians to choose case-by-case the best "ingredients" for a "successful recipe" (i.e., patient selection, interface, ventilator, etc.) and, in any case, if a NIV attempt fails, intubation must not be delayed [9]. This must be carefully considered, particularly in prehospital emergency care, where appropriate training of ambulance personnel, adequate infrastructure, and coordination with emergency departments are also key ingredients. This ensures that, if the response to NIV is good (improved patient's comfort, oxygenation, vital signs, respiratory rate, and work of breathing), the treatment is not interrupted at the arrival to the emergency department and, if progressive deterioration or intolerance to NIV therapy emerges, an alternative strategy is put in place as soon as possible [10].

6.2 Indications, Contraindications, and Patient Selection

6.2.1 Indications

Current NIV guidelines, which do not specifically focus on prehospital settings, tend to draw precise indications for subgroups of patients who can benefit most from NIV. Unfortunately, guidelines structured in this way are not easily applied to prehospital settings, where diagnostic tools are limited and other factors come into consideration [10].

The best candidate for NIV is an awake patient in respiratory distress who is alert and cooperative and has an intact gag reflex. In our opinion, once absolute contraindications have been ruled out, patients who can benefit from an early initiation of NIV are those with ARF and SpO_2 of 88–92% if with known COPD or < 92% if with other disorders, or signs of increased work of breathing and respiratory distress, such as nasal flaring, mouth breathing, recruitment of accessory and expiratory muscle, intercostal recession, paradoxical abdominal movement, tachypnea, tachycardia, hypertension or hypotension, and diaphoresis [11].

In prehospital settings, it is also appropriate using NIV to relief symptoms in patients with ARF and respiratory fatigue and do-not-intubate orders or when comorbidities, performance status, and prognosis are unknown at the time of intervention. Administering NIV while en route to the hospital gives time to explore the patient's wishes by communicating directly with him/her, or relatives, or family doctor, avoiding intubation or other invasive procedures that might reveal to be futile and burdensome [12, 13].

Inpatient studies suggest that COPD and CPE patients are those most likely to benefit from prehospital NIV [4].

6.2.2 Contraindications

Absolute contraindications are the same regardless of the setting: cardiac or respiratory arrest, extreme psychomotor agitation, severe hemodynamic instability, coma, multiple organ failure, airway obstruction, or inability to keep patent airway. Mild agitation or poor cooperation, upper gastrointestinal hemorrhage or vomiting, inability to expectorate copious secretions, recent frail upper gastrointestinal, or airway surgery, which are usually considered relative contraindications, need a more careful assessment in prehospital settings. Suspected pneumothoraxes should be treated prior to initiation of NIV therapy [14, 15].

6.3 Safety: NIV Vs. Orotracheal Intubation

NIV is generally safe, especially when the provider is able to evaluate the response to treatment and definitively secure patient's airway if respiratory collapse appears imminent.

NIV also has a lower rate of complications such as pneumonias, vocal injury, and tracheal stenosis than invasive techniques [16]. Intubation requires sedation and neuromuscular paralysis followed by admission to the intensive care unit. This is likely to result in recovery with worthwhile quality of life only if the patient's health and functional status were reasonable before the acute illness. Patients presenting with ARF who have severe underlying disease and multiple comorbidities may benefit less from intubation and invasive ventilation. NIV does not require sedation or neuromuscular paralysis and can be appropriately used in patients with relatively severe underlying disease [4].

It may appear logical that extensive use of advanced airway devices may solve several problems of ARF management, but numerous studies are not encouraging because prehospital setting is not an ideal scenario to perform endotracheal intubation or to use supraglottic devices for various reasons. First, the operator is often not in the optimal position for direct laryngoscopic visualization of the airway or to place a laryngeal mask. Second, the emergency setting and the frequent clinical instability of the patient represents stressor and distractors, which may severely compromise the performance of the operator. Third, frequently the operators lack adequate training in advanced airway management, which is not free of complications. Data on the rate of failed intubations vary among studies (ranging from 1% to 25%) considering events as tube misplacement, four or more intubation attempts, and failed intubation. Moreover, episodes hypoxemia with $SpO2 < 90\%$ have been reported during or immediately after intubation in 10–60% of cases, eventually triggering severe bradycardia in 20% [17].

6.4 Time Issue

An important issue regarding prehospital application of NIV is the additional time required to prepare the equipment and to fit the NIV-mask/helmet to the face/neck of the patient. This raises the question as to whether the extra effort associated with a prolonged on-scene time is justified, in particular when the ambulance transport time is short, as in most metropolitan areas. However, only a minimal additional time of about 6–7 min is required for a well-trained emergency team to apply NIV using a transport ventilator [14]. Furthermore, the time lag between the patient's arrival to the Emergency Department and the actual start of NIV therapy is most likely longer than the additional time spent in prehospital setting in order to initiate NIV. In conclusion, prehospital NIV-treatment could be a valuable option, even when the distance between the emergency scene and the hospital is short [18], in particular as far as CPE is concerned [19].

6.5 Modalities of NIV

The term NIV covers different forms of ventilatory support, which can be provided as continuous positive airway pressure (CPAP), continuous positive airway pressure supplemented by pressure support (PSV), or as positive pressure ventilation such as bi-level inspiratory positive airway pressure (BIPAP).

CPAP and PSV/BIPAP have different indications, but as far as the prehospital setting is concerned, CPAP should probably be considered as first line intervention, because it is cheap, can be administered without a ventilator and, most importantly, is easier to implement in clinical practice without long training [14, 15].

In the past, technology constrained the use of prehospital NIV. Limitations of using hospital NIV devices included size, cost, durability, and oxygen consumption. Nowadays, various devices are commercially available, but providers should be aware of differences in performance and design of Venturi flow generators.

6.5.1 CPAP

CPAP consists of the application of continuous positive pressure to the lung. However, it is of utmost importance to bear in mind that positive end-expiratory pressure (PEEP) is not the only parameter to consider. In fact, in order to minimize the work of breathing, airway pressure should not fluctuate during spontaneous breathing with CPAP. To obtain this, the airflow delivered by CPAP devices should always be higher than the patient's peak inspiratory flow so that a stable positive airway pressure is ensured during the entire breathing cycle. A minimum of 60 L/min is generally considered sufficient to guarantee a constant CPAP level under most degrees of inspiratory demand, although higher flows might be required in cases of severe respiratory distress and high minute ventilation [20].

6.5.1.1 Venturi-Type Flow Generator System

In prehospital settings, the best way to produce high-flow with the least compressed oxygen is by using a *Venturi-type flow generator system* that uses *Venturi's* effect to accelerate the gas coming from a cylinder mixing it with room air ensuring flow >60 L/min (until > 100 L/min). This allows to deliver oxygen at flow that surely overcomes patient's inspiratory demand, thereby ensuring a reduction of inspiratory effort and a constant level of positive airway pressure even at high level of respiratory distress. Moreover, the operator can regulate the level of PEEP with a dedicated expiratory valve regardless of inspiratory gas flow. The main drawback of every system based on Venturi's principle is that when flow is increased, FiO_2 is diminished because of the greater amount of room air entering the system. There are several commercially available devices for administering CPAP, each with slight differences in terms of characteristics and performance, so each user should be familiar with the devices available in his service [20].

6.5.1.2 Boussignac System

Another much less performing option to deliver CPAP is the *Boussignac system*, based on the positive pressure generated by the acceleration and collision of oxygen molecules passing through a cylinder with four micro-channels (virtual valve). This system has some limits. First, the actual FiO_2 inspired and PEEP generated critically depend on the gas flow reaching the Boussignac's valve, making the flow delivered by the cylinder the limitating element for FiO_2 and PEEP, which are mutually dependent. Second, the maximum positive pressure achieved with the Boussignac system is around 9 cm H_2O at an oxygen input flow of 30 L/min, which is far below the minimum of 60 L/min generally considered safe. Third, the system itself requires the patient breathing against the virtual valve to exhale, thus adding an additional expiratory work and making end expiratory pressure variable. Fourth, the inspiratory flow generated by a dyspnoic patient may exceed the mask flow, creating a negative pressure with large variability of airway pressure [20]. The Boussignac system has the advantages of being small, easy to place, and just requiring connection to oxygen cylinder, making it convenient for use by paramedical personnel on ambulances [21]. Additionally, for low maximal flow generated by the patient, it allows less mixing with room air, thus delivering higher FiO_2 than other CPAP/NIV systems, which makes it suitable in hypoxemic patients with not too high breathing frequency [20].

These CPAP devices are easily usable during ambulance transport; they do not require electrical power but only an oxygen source, making them ideal devices for prehospital emergency settings.

6.5.2 CPAP-ASB and BIPAP

CPAP-Assisted Spontaneous Breathing (CPAP-ASB) and Bi-level positive airway pressure (BiPAP) can only be administered by a ventilator.

In CPAP-ASB, when the patient starts the inspiratory effort, it triggers the ventilator to deliver inspiratory assistance with pressure support using a decelerated flow, which keeps the pressure constant. When the inspiratory flow descends below a preset percentage of its maximum value (usually 25–30%), the pressure support is discontinued, and the pressure drops down to the predetermined PEEP.

In BIPAP mode, two levels of pressure and the time each level lasts are set: P high and P low, T insp, T exp. In any moment the patient can breathe spontaneously.

6.5.2.1 Transport Ventilators

Ideally, a portable ventilator should be light-weighted, but robust, and use available gas or electrical supplies sparingly. There are several devices marketed as transport ventilators, but they can be divided in three main categories according to the technology used to provide ventilation. The first group includes pneumatic ventilators using compressed oxygen, the second and third electrically powered ventilators using turbine and compressor or piston, respectively [21].

From a practical point of view, there are major differences among transport ventilators in terms of general characteristics and technical reliability. They differ for oxygen consumption, and battery duration, determined both by battery type and ventilator settings. Unless an adapter is used for power supply from the vehicle, batteries should be available to provide sufficient power for the duration of transport, including possible delays. Turbine-driven ventilators require more power, and this must be considered. Most transport ventilators are able to maintain adequate PEEP and pressure support, even in the presence of minimal to moderate leak. However, some devices cannot provide adequate pressurization with <18% pressure support delivered. Leaks, which are not uncommon during transport, may increase the patient's effort and asynchrony with the ventilator. Other characteristics such as triggering delay, i.e., time between onset of airway pressure decay and flow delivery, and patient effort to trigger, i.e., pressure-time product per cycle, can vary among different devices. This is important because triggering and leak compensation performance are crucial issues while performing non-invasive ventilation [21, 22]. The consequence of patient-ventilator asynchrony (double triggering, ineffective triggering, etc.), mostly due to poor ventilator setup, could be an increase in the work of breathing due to the patient fighting the ventilator and worsen the situation [23].

Turbine-driven models outperform gas-driven ventilators in tidal volume accuracy, triggering characteristics, and pressurization performance, with performance similar to ICU ventilators in pressure support mode (better tidal volume delivery and trigger sensitivity) [24].

However uncommon, failure of portable ventilators may occur and, when it happens, cannot be fixed quickly or easily. Thus, a tool for manual ventilation must always be immediately available.

The efficiency of devices in terms of oxygen consumption is an important topic, especially in prehospital use, for oxygen availability on ambulances is limited and transportation time may vary greatly. Furthermore, ambulances in some countries have oxygen sources that can generally deliver only up to a maximum of 15 L/min. Therefore, when higher oxygen flows are needed, as with the Boussignac CPAP system, it is necessary to use two tanks simultaneously to achieve a gas delivery of 30 L/min [20]. Modern ventilators consume gas not only for supplying the patient's minute ventilation, but also for providing background rate of gas flow (bias flow) through the breathing circuit, or to control the ventilator cycle itself. If gas consumption is not displayed by the ventilator, a crude estimate can be made. Provisions for patient deterioration should be made when predicting FiO_2. The oxygen requirement for transfer includes an additional 50% in case of unforeseen delays.

$$\text{Gas consumption} = \left(\text{minute ventilation} + \text{bias flow}\right) \times \left[\left(Fi_{O2} - 0.2\right)/0.8\right] + \text{cycling requirement} \tag{6.1}$$

A more accurate approximation can be obtained using [22]:

$$\text{Gas consumption} = \left[\text{minute volume} + \left(\text{bias flow} \times \left[Ti/Ti+Te\right]\right)\right] \times \left[\left(Fi_{O2} - 0.2\right)/0.8\right] + \text{cycling requirement} \tag{6.2}$$

Given the lack of space in the back of an ambulance or helicopter, the number of cylinders that can be carried is limited; hence the number needed to complete the journey must be carefully calculated prior to embarking. There are also nomograms to estimate the duration of oxygen cylinders, even with a number of limitations. For example, during air flights, pressure differentials can cause a reduction in ventilator consumption for a set minute volume. Local variations in temperature can also affect consumption. Furthermore, apart from oxygen and battery consumption, when using transport ventilators there is a logistical issue of space on and around the bed. The more equipment is involved, the less space the clinicians have to access the patient (some ventilators may be much more cumbersome than a venturimeter).

Gas Cylinder
A gas cylinder is a containment apparatus that will store a gaseous compound under pressure for use in medical settings. The physical form of the stored compound can be gas and/or liquid, with the ultimate output from the apparatus being gaseous. Gas cylinders are labeled from A to M, with increasing volume as the letters of the alphabet proceeds. E-sized cylinders are the most commonly used size in medical settings. E cylinders have a service pressure of 1900 psi, but may be filled up to 10% more to 2200 psi.

Use Boyle's law to calculate how much oxygen time is remaining in an E-sized cylinder. Boyle's law states that at a fixed temperature (room temperature) of an ideal gas, the pressure is inversely proportional to volume. Boyle's law can be further rearranged to state that pressure times volume is equal to a constant. The following is the formula:

$$P1^* V1 = P2^* V2 \quad (6.3)$$

One could compare a cylinder of gas at filled volume (V1 = 660 L) and pressure (P1 = 2200 psi) to the current pressure (P2) read on the cylinder. This would provide the information needed to solve for the current volume (V2) remaining in the tank in liters. The following is the formula:

$$P1 / P2^* V1 = V2 \quad (6.4)$$

or this Volume (V2) can be used to determine the amount of unit time remaining left on the cylinder, given a current flow rate of the gas:

V2 / Flow rate = unit time remaining

or Liters of oxygen remaining in the tank/oxygen setting in liters/minute = Minutes of oxygen remaining.

6.6 NIV Interfaces

Different interfaces (Table 6.1) are available for administration of NIV. Choosing the appropriate interface for patients with ARF involves consideration of patient preferences and tolerance and determining the correct size and fit [25].

6.6.1 Helmet Vs. Masks

As mouth breathing is prevalent in patients with ARF, a face mask (oro-nasal or total face mask) is considered more suitable and effective interface than nasal mask. On the other hand, the helmet has the advantage of avoiding skin contact, hence improving patient tolerance independent of face morphology [25]. Masks can create problems of discomfort ranging from claustrophobia to pain on pressure points (all factors that can worsen the efficacy of the device, thus reducing patient's compliance) beside fitting problems (for example in edentulous patients) [26–28]. Helmets are surely more comfortable to fit, allow clearance of secretions and interaction with caregivers, and are better tolerated than face masks [25]. If a facemask is used, it is important to keep in mind that securing the interface too tightly decreases patient's tolerance and increases the risk of facial skin damage; therefore, when the headgear is fixed, it should be possible to allow two fingers beneath it (the so called, 2-finger rule).

It has recently been suggested that in subjects on NIV with non-hypercapnic ARF, the use of helmet could reduce intubation rate and hospital mortality than a face mask or a nasal mask [25, 29, 30]. However, on the need of shifting to advanced airway management, helmet removal may delay the airway access more than mask [20, 26]; thus, the use of helmet can be recommended if provided with a zip closure to avoid dangerous delays in the management of upper airways.

Helmet allows significantly higher levels of PEEP sustained throughout NIV therapy, which results in a significant reduction of breathing frequency and similar oxygen saturation levels on lower FiO2 than with face-mask [25, 29, 30]. On the other hand, the ability to generate higher PEEP (surely useful in terms of alveolar recruitment and improvement of gas exchange) may increase the rate of complications hard to manage in limited resource settings. Among these are worsening of hemodynamics in hypovolemic patients or with right ventricular failure, new onset or worsening of pneumothorax, gastric distention, and aspiration [20, 26].

Helmet has less air leakage due to its lack of contact with the face and a better seal around the neck, which allows titration to higher positive airway pressures without substantial air leakage [25, 29, 30].

There has been always a concern that a helmet may increase dead space, thus increasing $PaCO_2$ as a result of its large internal volume and high compliance, which may in turn lead to CO_2 rebreathing. In order to prevent CO_2 rebreathing, a flow output of at least 60 L/min is necessary

Table 6.1 NIV interfaces

Interface	Description
Nasal mask	Nose only and rests on the upper lip, the sides of the nose, and the nasal bridge
Oro-nasal mask (also referred to as a face mask)	Nose and mouth and rests on the chin, the sides of the nose and mouth, and the nasal bridge
Nasal pillow mask	On the rim of the nostrils (mainly in stable patients with sleep-disordered breathing)
Oral mask	Inside the mouth between the teeth and lips and has a tongue guide to prevent the tongue from obstructing the airway passage (not common in practice)
Total face mask	The whole face
Helmet CPAP	A transparent hood that covers the entire head and face of the patient and has a rubber collar neck seal

when using helmet to perform CPAP, but this may create problem of cylinder depletion unless high efficiency Venturi systems are used to reduce oxygen consumption [20].

Interfaces used for PSV have been shown to affect patient–ventilator interaction. Of all interfaces, the helmet creates more problems with patient–ventilator synchrony and ventilator cycling due to its soft compliant wall, upward displacement, and elevated internal compressible volume [25]. To avoid these problems, a helmet designed to deliver pressure support should be used (less internal volume, lower compliance with an inflatable collar neck, assuring less upward displacement). In addition, it is important to increase both pressure support level and PEEP and to use the highest pressurization rate [25].

For these reasons, the use of inspiratory support, surely useful in hypercapnic ARF, needs a higher level of training of prehospital staff compared to CPAP, beginning from adequate selection of devices and interfaces to deep knowledge of patient-to-ventilator interactions. In prehospital emergency care, helmet CPAP is probably the most efficient and practical choice to administer NIV even by a minimally trained crew. A practical way to check if pressure in the CPAP helmet is above the PEEP throughout the respiratory cycle is to check that gas flow through the expiratory valve is always present [31].

6.6.2 High Flow Nasal Cannula (HFNC)

It is possible that in the near future another interface that has been increasingly used in patients with ARF with satisfactory results will be implemented in prehospital settings as well: HFNC [32].

This may appear attractive for the ease of positioning and setting of devices, as well as for the comfort of the patient and the ease of access to airway (these devices may remain in place ensuring preoxygenation and apneic oxygenation) [33]. However, there are some limitations to be considered: first, these devices need portable power supply for turbine and humidifier, which may be too cumbersome; if this is not available, treatment discontinuation may occur in case of delay in transportation from rescue place to emergency room [34]. Second, although these devices can ensure CO_2 washout from upper airways, thus reducing anatomical dead space, they lose efficacy in highly tachypnoic patients breathing with open mouth. Moreover, the level of pressure ensured by the devices is useful to keep upper airways open but not effective for alveolar recruitment. Manufacturers claim a PEEP level of 1 cmH2O every 10 L of delivered flow, up to a maximum of 6 cmH2O; some studies found maximal PEEP levels around 3 cmH2O, with substantial reductions in case of open mouth breathing (https://rebelem.com/high-flow-nasal-cannula-hfnc-part-1-how-it-works/). So far, most of the studies on HFNC are from countries where this method has been introduced for interhospital transport of critically ill children [32]. The Prehospital High-Flow Nasal Oxygen Therapy (PRHOXY-1) is an ongoing single-center, open-label, parallel, randomized trial with 1:2 allocation ratio (two patients assigned to standard oxygen therapy for each patient assigned to High Flow Nasal Oxygen therapy) (ClinicalTrials.gov Identifier: NCT03326830). The purpose is comparing oxygen therapy by HFNC, initiated in the prehospital setting in patients with ARF, with standard oxygen therapy, in terms of oxygenation at arrival to the hospital and need of mechanical ventilation during the subsequent 28 days [35].

6.7 Cost-Effectiveness

Prehospital treatment of ARF has substantial knock-on costs for the health service. Patients with life-threatening respiratory illness often require prolonged hospital stay and/or critical care, owing to the need of ventilatory support, which may be greater in case of inadequate or inappropriate initial management. Conversely, appropriate use of early intervention can reduce the need for intubation and ventilation, thus reducing critical care costs [4].It is unclear whether there is enough evidence justifying extensive use of prehospital NIV. This is generally used in hospitals, but it may be more effective if started prior to hospital arrival; nevertheless, its use for respiratory failure in prehospital settings remains limited for the following reasons:

- Prehospital and in-hospital settings differ in a number of ways, which makes the findings of the latter difficult to extrapolate to the former.
- The initial assessment of patients is limited by the difficulty in conducting a full clinical examination and by the absence of diagnostic investigations, which creates less certainty about underlying disease in prehospital settings16.

- The equipment available is limited by space constraints in ambulance.

Prehospital NIV has been evaluated in a number of trials [36–45] and it seems to reduce mortality and intubation rates, but these trials were small and findings were not consistent.

These evidences of effectiveness would not justify an implementation of prehospital NIV because the cost of such implementation could be substantial and could represent poor value for health care if associated with a small health benefits or prehospital NIV was applied only to a small number of patients. Implementing prehospital NIV would require additional training for many paramedics and additional equipment for many ambulances. The substantial costs associated with these interventions require a more robust evidence of clinical effectiveness prior to implementation.

Consequently, an economic analysis is required to determine the cost/effectiveness of prehospital NIV compared with standard usual care for ARF [4].

The advantages of prehospital NIV over conventional management include reduced breathlessness, improved arterial blood gases, decreased intubation rates, mortality, morbidity, and in-hospital length of stay. All these advantages would possibly translate in reduced health care costs [46].

Furthermore, NIV is associated with higher success rate in weaning from invasive mechanical ventilation, because it allows voluntary coughing, reduces the need for sedation and muscle relaxants, and supports self-feeding and communication [47]. In addition, the training required to deliver NIV is less extensive than the training required for endotracheal intubation.

When ARF is associated with elevated carbon dioxide levels and acidosis, BiPAP can improve gas exchange and outcome and may be more efficient than endotracheal intubation and controlled mechanical ventilation for it matches the patient's spontaneous respiratory drive; in fact, in these circumstances oxygen therapy may reduce respiratory drive and worsen hypercapnia and thus outcome [48].

In addition, it seems that NIV is more likely to be effective if used early in the course of respiratory failure, before breathing fatigue develops [4]. This raises the possibility that prehospital NIV could be more effective than in-hospital NIV.

6.8 Conclusions

Acute respiratory distress is a common diagnostic dilemma for paramedics and can be due to various conditions. The goals of care include identifying the cause, promptly initiating targeted management, stabilizing the airway, and observing for ventilatory improvement or deterioration [49].

In patients with severe respiratory distress, prehospital NIV has been shown to reduce the need for intubation or mechanical ventilation upon admission to a hospital as well as in hospital mortality.

NIV is generally safe if the providers are skilled.

Nevertheless, the available evidence of advantages of pre/hospital NIV is still limited.

Further evidence on feasibility, clinical effectiveness, and cost-effectiveness is therefore required before implementation of prehospital CPAP can be recommended.

In summary, essential prerequisites for a successful out-of-hospital use of NIV are special training programs for Emergency Physicians to guarantee not only a correct administration of the therapy, but also an optimal selection of patients, which remains one of the main challenges.

References

1. Parshall MB, et al. An official American thoracic society statement: update on the mechanisms, assessment, and management of dyspnea. Am J Respir Crit Care Med. 2012;185(4):435–52. https://doi.org/10.1164/rccm.201111-2042ST.
2. Laribi S, et al. Epidemiology of patients presenting with dyspnea to emergency departments in Europe and the Asia-Pacific region. Eur J Emerg Med. 2019;26(5):345–9. https://doi.org/10.1097/MEJ.0000000000000571.

3. Prekker ME, et al. The epidemiology and outcome of prehospital respiratory distress. Acad Emerg Med. 2014;21(5):543–50. https://doi.org/10.1111/acem.12380.

4. Pandor A, et al. Pre-hospital non-invasive ventilation for acute respiratory failure: a systematic review and cost-effectiveness evaluation. Health Technol Assess. 2015;19(42) v–vi:1–102. https://doi.org/10.3310/hta19420.

5. Baudouin S, Blumenthal S, Cooper B, Davidson C, Davison A, Elliott M, et al. Non-invasive ventilation in acute respiratory failure –British thoracic society standards of care committee. Thorax. 2002;57:192–211.

6. Maio RF, Garrison HG, Spaite DW, Desmond JS, Gregor MA, Cayten CG, Chew JL Jr, Hill EM, Joyce SM, MacKenzie EJ, et al. Emergency medical services outcomes project I (EMSOP I): prioritizing conditions for outcomes research. Ann Emerg Med. 1999;33(4):423–32.

7. Nicholl J, West J, Goodacre S, Turner J. The relationship between distance to hospital and patient mortality in emergencies: an observational study. Emerg Med J. 2007;24(9):665–8.

8. Wang HE, Davis DP, O'Connor RE, Domeier RM. Drug-assisted intubation in the prehospital setting (resource document to NAEMSP position statement). Prehosp Emerg Care. 2006;10(2):261–71. https://doi.org/10.1080/10903120500541506.

9. Scala R, Pisani L. Noninvasive ventilation in acute respiratory failure: which recipe for success? Eur Respir Rev. 2018;27:180029. https://doi.org/10.1183/16000617.0029-2018.

10. Rochwerg B, Brochard L, Elliott MW, et al. Official ERS/ATS clinical practice guidelines: noninvasive ventilation for acute respiratory failure. Eur Respir J. 2017;50:1602426. https://doi.org/10.1183/13993003.02426-2016.

11. Fuller GW, et al. The ACUTE (ambulance CPAP: use, treatment effect and economics) feasibility study: a pilot randomised controlled trial of pre-hospital CPAP for acute respiratory failure. Pilot Feasibility Stud. 2018;4:86. https://doi.org/10.1186/s40814-018-0281-9.

12. Garuti G, et al. Out-of-hospital helmet CPAP in acute respiratory failure reduces mortality: a study led by nurses. Monaldi Arch Chest Dis. 2010;73(4):145–51. https://doi.org/10.4081/monaldi.2010.283.

13. Thompson J, et al. Out-of-hospital continuous positive airway pressure ventilation versus usual care in acute respiratory failure: a randomized controlled trial. Ann Emerg Med. 2008;52(3):232–41., 241.e1. https://doi.org/10.1016/j.annemergmed.2008.01.006.

14. Hensel M, et al. Prehospital non-invasive ventilation in acute respiratory failure is justified even if the distance to hospital is short. Am J Emerg Med. 2019;37(4):651–6. https://doi.org/10.1016/j.ajem.2018.07.001.

15. Masip J, et al. Indications and practical approach to non-invasive ventilation in acute heart failure. Eur Heart J. 2018;39:17–25. https://doi.org/10.1093/eurheartj/ehx580.

16. Sullivan CE, Issa FG, Berthon-Jones M, Eves L. Reversal of obstructive sleep apnoea by continuous positive airway pressure applied through the nares. Lancet. 1981;1(8225):862–5. https://doi.org/10.1016/s0140-6736(81)92140-1.

17. Gnugnoli DM, Singh A, Shafer K. EMS Field Intubation. StatPearls; 2021.

18. Mazen J, Sayed E, et al. Impact of prehospital mechanical ventilation. A retrospective matched cohort study of 911 calls in the United States. Medicine (Baltimore). 2019;98(4):e13990. https://doi.org/10.1097/MD.0000000000013990.

19. Plaisance P, et al. A randomized study of out-of-hospital continuous positive airway pressure for acute cardiogenic pulmonary oedema: physiological and clinical effects. Eur Heart J. 2007;28:2895–901. https://doi.org/10.1093/eurheartj/ehm502.

20. Brusasco, et al. CPAP devices for emergency prehospital use: a bench study. Respir Care. 2015;60(12):1777–85. https://doi.org/10.4187/respcare.04134.

21. L'Her E, et al. Bench-test comparison of 26 emergency and transport ventilators. Crit Care. 2014;18:506. http://ccforum.com/content/18/5/506

22. Fludger S, FRCA MBCBBS(H), Klein A, FRCA MBBS. Portable ventilators. Contin Educ Anaesth Crit Care Pain. 2008;8(6):199–203. https://doi.org/10.1093/bjaceaccp/mkn039.

23. MacIntyre NR, et al. Physiologic effects of noninvasive ventilation. Respir Care. 2019;64(6):617–28. https://doi.org/10.4187/respcare.06635.

24. Holets SR, Davies JD. Should a portable ventilator be used in all in-hospital transports? Respir Care. 2016;61(6):839–53. https://doi.org/10.4187/respcare.04745.

25. BaHammam AS, Deep Singh T, Gupta R, Pandi-Perumal SR. Choosing the proper interface for positive airway pressure therapy in subjects with acute respiratory failure. Respir Care. 2018;63(2):227–37. https://doi.org/10.4187/respcare.05787.

26. Gay PC, et al. Complications of noninvasive ventilation in acute care. Respir Care. 2009;54(2):246–57.

27. Rodriguez E, et al. Clinical review: helmet and non-invasive mechanical ventilation in critically ill patients. Crit Care. 2013;17:223. http://ccforum.com/content/17/2/223

28. Dilken O, et al. Noninvasive ventilation: challenges and pitfalls. EMJ Respir. 2018;6(1):100–8.

29. Patel BK, Wolfe KS, Pohlman AS, Hall JB, Kress JP. Effect of noninvasive ventilation delivered by helmet vs face mask on the rate of endotracheal intubation in patients with acute respiratory distress syndrome: a randomized clinical trial. JAMA. 2016;315(22):2435–41. https://doi.org/10.1001/jama.2016.6338.

30. Tatham KC, Ko M, Palozzi L, et al. Helmet interface increases lung volumes at equivalent ventilator pressures compared to the face mask interface during non-

invasive ventilation. Crit Care. 2020;24:504. https://doi.org/10.1186/s13054-020-03216-7.

31. Foti G, et al. Is helmet CPAP first line pre-hospital treatment of presumed severe acute pulmonary edema? Intensive Care Med. 2009;35(4):656–62. https://doi.org/10.1007/s00134-008-1354-7.

32. Schlapbach LJ, et al. High-flow nasal cannula (HFNC) support in interhospital transport of critically ill children. Intensive Care Med. 2014;40(4):592–9. https://doi.org/10.1007/s00134-014-3226-7.

33. Drake MG, et al. High-flow nasal cannula oxygen in adults: an evidence-based assessment. Ann Am Thorac Soc. 2018;15(2):145–55. https://doi.org/10.1513/AnnalsATS.201707-548FR.

34. Díaz-Lobato S, Perales JMC, et al. Things to keep in mind in high flow therapy: as usual the devil is in the detail. Int J Crit Care Emerg Med. 2018;4:048. https://doi.org/10.23937/2474-3674/1510048.

35. Mauri T, Alban L, Turrini C, et al. Optimum support by high-flow nasal cannula in acute hypoxemic respiratory failure: effects of increasing flow rates. Intensive Care Med. 2017;43:1453.

36. Austin MA, Wills KE. Effect of continuous positive airway pressure on mortality in the treatment of acute cardiogenic pulmonary edema in the prehospital setting: randomized controlled trial. Acad Emerg Med. 2012;19(Suppl. 1):283(abstract 534).

37. Ducros L, Logeart D, Vicaut E, Henry P, Plaisance P, Collet JP, et al. CPAP for acute cardiogenic pulmonary oedema from out-of-hospital to cardiac intensive care unit: a randomised multicentre study. Intensive Care Med. 2011;37:1501–9. https://doi.org/10.1007/s00134-011-2311-4.

38. Frontin P, Bounes V, Houze-Cerfon CH, Charpentier S, Houze-Cerfon V, Ducasse JL. Continuous positive airway pressure for cardiogenic pulmonary edema: a randomized study. Am J Emerg Med. 2011;29:775–81. https://doi.org/10.1016/j.ajem.2010.03.007.

39. Mas A, Alonso G, Perez C, Saura P, Alcoverro JM, Guirado M. Non-invasive mechanical ventilation for acute dyspnea in out-of-hospital emergency care. Intensive Care Med. 2002;28:S69 (abstract 256).

40. Plaisance P, Pirracchio R, Berton C, Vicaut E, Payen D. A randomized study of out-of-hospital continuous positive airway pressure for acute cardiogenic pulmonary oedema: physiological and clinical effects. Eur Heart J. 2007;28:2895–901. https://doi.org/10.1093/eurheartj/ehm502.

41. Roessler MS, Schmid DS, Michels P, Schmid O, Jung K, Stober J, et al. Early out-of-hospital non-invasive ventilation is superior to standard medical treatment in patients with acute respiratory failure: a pilot study. Emerg Med J. 2012;29:409–14. https://doi.org/10.1136/emj.2010.106393.

42. Schmidbauer W, Ahlers O, Spies C, Dreyer A, Mager G, Kerner T. Early prehospital use of non-invasive ventilation improves acute respiratory failure in acute exacerbation of chronic obstructive pulmonary disease. Emerg Med J. 2011;28:626–7. https://doi.org/10.1136/emj.2009.089102.

43. Thompson J, Petrie DA, Ackroyd-Stolarz S, Bardua DJ. Out-of-hospital continuous positive airway pressure ventilation versus usual care in acute respiratory failure: a randomized controlled trial. Ann Emerg Med. 2008;52:232–41. https://doi.org/10.1016/j.annemergmed.2008.01.006.

44. Craven RA, Singletary N, Bosken L, Sewell E, Payne M, Lipsey R. Use of bilevel positive airway pressure in out-of-hospital patients. Acad Emerg Med. 2000;7:1065–8. https://doi.org/10.1111/j.1553-2712.2000.tb02102.x.

45. Weitz G, Struck J, Zonak A, Balnus S, Perras B, Dodt C. Prehospital noninvasive pressure support ventilation for acute cardiogenic pulmonary edema. Eur J Emerg Med. 2007;14:276–9. https://doi.org/10.1097/MEJ.0b013e32826fb377.

46. Sinuff T, Cook DJ, Hill NS. Does noninvasive positive pressure ventilation improve outcome in acute hypoxemic respiratory failure? A systematic review. Crit Care Med. 2004;32:2516.

47. Devlin JW, Nava S, Fong JJ, Bahhady I, Hill NS. Survey of sedation practices during noninvasive positive-pressure ventilation to treat acute respiratory failure. Crit Care Med. 2007;35(10):2298–302.

48. Daily JC, Wang HE. Noninvasive positive pressure ventilation: resource document for the national association of EMS physicians position statement. Prehosp Emerg Care. 2011;15(3):432–8. https://doi.org/10.3109/10903127.2011.569851.

49. Mal S, McLeod S, Iansavichene A, Dukelow A, Lewell M. Effect of out-of-hospital noninva-sive positive-pressure support ventilation in adult patients with severe respiratory distress: a systematic review and meta-analysis. Ann Emerg Med. 2014;63(5):600–7. e601

Current Strategies and Equipment for Non-invasive Ventilation in Emergency Medicine

Romina Peroné

Contents

7.1   Introduction

Heart failure is one of the leading causes of hospital admission in the world. The patients may develop shortness of breath and leg swelling rapidly over a few hours until the onset of pulmonary edema.

Acute cardiogenic pulmonary edema (ACPE) and Acute exacerbations of chronic obstructive pulmonary disease (COPD) are common causes of acute respiratory failure (ARF) in patients presenting to the emergency department.

ACPE is caused by left ventricular failure with elevated left ventricular filling pressure. Elevated filling pressure produces increases of the pressure in the pulmonary vessels and fluid extravasation into alveoli due to no reabsorption in lymphatic vessels. Pulmonary edema fluid can dilute surfactant, collapse in the alveoli causing a reduction in lung compliance, and increase work of breathing. Moreover, edema accumulates at the lung bases, causing mismatch of ventilation-perfusion with pathologic shunt formation and hypoxia [1].

The main therapeutic targets for patients with ACPE are the improvement of hypoxemia and respiratory distress.

The mainstay of treatment of this condition is the use of loop diuretics and vasodilators with supplemental oxygen.

From many years, Non-Invasive Positive Pressure Ventilation (NPPV) has been used as a support to medical therapy.

The NPPV refers to the administration of mechanical ventilation without using an invasive airway (endotracheal or tracheostomy tube); it can be provided in the form of continuous positive airway pressure (CPAP) and Bilevel mode using face or nasal mask.

The rationale for applying NPPV is to improve in the both conditions the cardiovascular and

R. Peroné (✉)
Anesthesiology Department, Pineta Grande Hospital,
Castelvolturno, Italy
e-mail: r.perone3@studenti.unisa.it

© The Author(s), under exclusive license to Springer Nature Switzerland AG 2023
G. Servillo, M. Vargas (eds.), *Non-invasive Mechanical Ventilation in Critical Care, Anesthesiology and Palliative Care*, https://doi.org/10.1007/978-3-031-36510-2_7

respiratory system, decreasing the venous return in right side of the heart and the left ventricle preload, transmural pressure, and relative afterload are also decreased.

Extrinsically applied positive end-expiratory pressure (ePRRP) increases alveolar size; the recruitment of collapsed alveoli reduces intrapulmonary shunt, improving lung compliance and decreasing the work of breathing [3, 4]. (Table 7.1)

The COPD is a chronic inflammatory lung disease that causes obstructed airflow from the lung with the collapse of small and medium-sized airways and mucus hypersecretion [6].

Table 7.1 Effects on the cardiovascular system

	Mechanism	Effect
Direct effects from PEEP	• Decreases LV afterload • Decreases LV diameter, leading to decreased MR	• LV unloading • Improved cardiac output
	• Increases transmural pressure	• Improved cardiac output
	• Increases Palv at the end of expiration	• Improved compliance (i.e., prevention of alveolar collapse)
Effects from or on gas exchange	• Reverses hypoxic vasoconstriction	• Lower RV afterload
	• Decreases in preload	• Improved pulmonary congestion
	• Improves ventilation/ perfusion matching	• Improved oxygenation
Effects from ventilatory support	• Improves work of breathing	• Improved tissue perfusion • Decreased myocardial consumption of oxygen
	• Improves hypercarbia and acidosis	• Improved RV afterload
Systemic effects	• Optimizes gas exchange, hence oxygenation and tissue perfusion	• Improved metabolic demand and peripheral perfusion

Symptoms include breathing difficulty, cough, mucus production, and wheezing.

COPD has an high mortality rate—up to 33% of patients admitted to the hospital who died despite appropriate therapy [5].

The COPD is typically associated with abnormalities of pulmonary gas exchange, ventilation/perfusion ratio mismatch, dynamic hyperinflation, increased peripheral resistance, and fatigue of the respiratory muscles, with development of hypercapnia (PaCO2 > 45 mmHg) and respiratory acidosis (pH > 7.35) [7].

The mainstay of treatment of patients includes bronchodilators, systemic steroids, antibiotics, and oxygen. When these measures fail, the patients are intubated with high mortality rate.

According to the Global Initiative for Chronic obstruction lung disease (GOCD) 2017 report, the NPPV is considered the first line intervention with standard medical therapy, improving lung pulmonary gas exchange by supporting alveolar ventilation, improving V/Q mismatch, and discharging the work of the respiratory muscles [2].

The NPPV is the first line treatment for acute respiratory distress in emergency department. The wide diffusion in emergency department finds explanations for the increasing longevity of the patients in many populations, for the increase in number of patients with comorbidities, most often on long-term oxygen therapy, and for the lack of beds in intensive care; furthermore, the technological evolution has produced ventilator with increased performance and more comfortable interfaces for the patients.

The NPPV avoids the endotracheal intubation, reducing the risk of adverse events, such as nosocomial infections, tracheal injury, and prolonged hospital length of stay [8].

7.2 State of Art

The use of NPPV to treat acute respiratory failure (ARF) has expanded enormously over the world in the past two decades.

Since the increased clinical use of NPPV in the 1980s, many studies have evaluated NPPV's effectiveness for pulmonary edema as reported in the early results of NAVA's studies. These works while demonstrating the effectiveness of the method on a clinical level, with the improvement of gas exchange and the reduction of endotracheal intubation, also reported [9] an increase in the incidence of myocardial infarction in the use of NPPV at two pressure levels compared to CPAP.

One study by Mehta and colleagues was terminated prematurely because of an excess number of patients with acute MI in the NPPV arm; in reality, the same author in a subsequent meta-analysis recognized mistake in the enrolling patients' protocol [10] and confirmed any relationship between NIPPV and MI rate, because the first cause of the pulmonary edema was the onset of MI.

One study of Gray [11] in 2008 on 1069 patients compared CPAP and BiPAP therapy with standard oxygen therapy in edema, concluding that the NPPV induced more improvements in respiratory distress and metabolic disturbance than that of standard oxygen therapy, but had no effect on short-term mortality.

In contrast, two subsequent meta-analyses reported best mortality rate and best intubation rates with NPPV use in the treatment of edema, but they also pointed out the attention about the small number of trials and about the variability of the definition and severity of edema [12–14].

Positive conclusions were confirmed in 2013 in an update of a meta-analysis in Cochrane [17] in 2008, with evaluation of 31 trials for a total of 2916 patients, with evidence of a significant reduction in short-term mortality with the use of NPPV in the treatment of the patients with pulmonary edema.

Current heart failure guidelines differ in their recommendations.

Canadian [13] and Australian guidelines [15] recommend the use of NIVV in the treatment of pulmonary edema in the absence of shock or persistent hypoxia and warn of the clinical risks of NPPV, including pnx, aspiration, and worsening of the hypercapnia.

In contrast, European guidelines [7] suggest to start early NPPV in patients who present tachypnea (respiratory rate greater than 25 breaths a minute) and hypoxia (SpO_2 less than 90%).

American guidelines [16] do not provide treatment guidance for edema.

The British Thoracic Society reiterates the need to use CPAP in edema, reserving bilevel mode if there is coexisting hypercapnia.

7.3 Discussion

The key to the success of NPPV in department of emergency depends on numerous factors, including the type and severity of ARF, patient selection, the patient compliance, the need to develop specific protocols (NPPV trial), appropriate methods patient's monitoring, and the expertise of the team.

There are two types of NPPV; the first mode is CPAP that applies a single pressure during all phases of the respiratory cycle, inspiration, and expiration. CPAP is a most useful modality for those patients with hypoxemic respiratory failure; it is analogous to positive end-expiratory pressure (PEEP) during mechanical ventilation.

The BiPAP modality delivers two levels of pressure to the patient: inspiratory positive airway pressure (IPAP) and expiratory positive airway pressure (EPAP); it can be used for patients with both hypercapnic and hypoxic respiratory failure.

When positive pressure is applied, the work of breathing can decrease by 60% through several different mechanisms [18].

The selection of the NPPV mode primarily depends on the clinical indication. BPAP remains a valid option for all disease states, and CPAP remains an highly effective therapy for patients with edema. The clinical indication remains a strong predictor of therapy success [19]. (Table 7.2)

Interfaces are devices that connect the ventilator tubing to the patient's face. There are many different types of interface, nasal, oronasal mask, full face, and helmets. Helmet interface encompassed the entire head often causing claustrophobia and anxiety, but it does not cause skin lesions and decreased air leak compared with the face mask interfaces.

Air leak is a typical feature of NPPV. Many modern ventilators can compensate for a large amount of air leak. Patient and ventilator synchrony is the key for NPPV success. There are numerous types of desynchrony: ineffective triggering, double triggering, auto triggering, premature cycle, and delayed cycling.

Ineffective triggering may occur when the sensitivity of the trigger is set too high, may also be secondary to high intrinsic PEEP, weakness of the patient.

Double triggering can be identified by two rapidly delivered breaths and may be the result of too short inspiratory time and too low inspiratory flow and tidal volume and cough.

Auto triggering takes place when the ventilator is triggered in a way other than the patient's respiratory effort.

Patient-ventilator asynchrony may be prevented by the optimization of setting ventilator using the screen ventilator waveforms, adjusting trigger sensitivity, modifying PEEP at the right level, and minimizing air leak.

Emergency physicians should be confident with device they use and choose the appropriate mask for increasing patient comfort and avoid to stop the therapy.

The ability of ICU physicians to detect the major patient–ventilator asynchronies during invasive ventilation by visual inspection of flow and pressure waveforms, as displayed on the ventilator screen, is the main indicator of the success of therapy [20]. (Table 7.3)

Patients' intolerance of non-invasive ventilation can be reduced by training of the patient before the application with clear explanation and reassurance, using special cautious analgosedation. Hypoxic and hypercapnic effects on mental status may be in part responsible for this intolerance.

Table 7.2 Type of evidence in certain disease

Type of evidence	Disease
Strong	ACPE
	COPD
	Weaning in COPD patient
Intermediate	Preoxygenation in hypoxemic Respiratory failure
	Post-extubation respiratory failure
Weak	ALI/ARDS
	Status asthmaticus
	Pneumonia

Table 7.3 Waveform

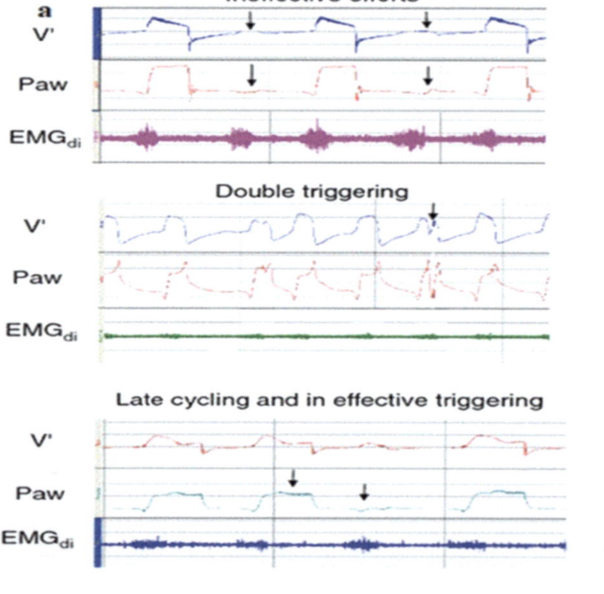

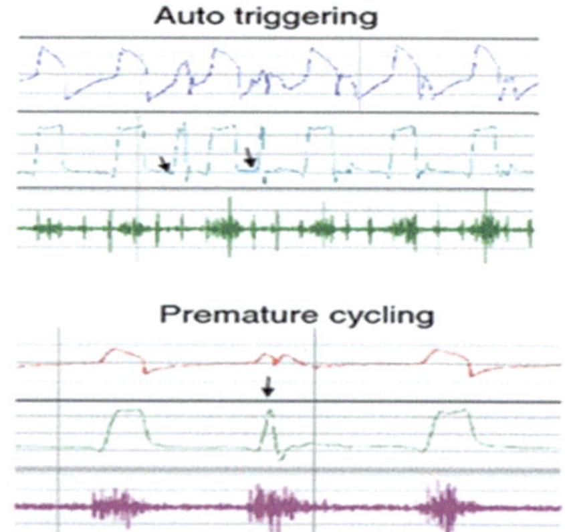

Table 7.4 Monitoring the efficacy of NPPV

Subjective parameters	Objective parameters
Mental status change	Heart rate
Patient-ventilator asynchrony	Respiratory rate
Accessory muscle use	Arterial blood gas
Patient comfort	Oxygen saturation
The degree of dyspnea	Blood pressure
Physical examination	Expiratory capnography transcut

Contraindication to NPPV is the need of airway protection because of altered mental status, uncooperative patient, hemodynamic instability, aspiration risk, and facial deformities because of pathology or trauma.

A common practice is to begin with 5 cm H_2O. PEEP that can be titrated every 10–15 min by increasing pressure by 2 cm H_2O with a goal of improving the SpO_2 or PaO_2,because a rapid titration could result in hypotension. Inspiratory pressure is set using the IPAP or PS, IPAP setting 12–15 cm H_2O.

The peak inspiratory pressure suggests an approach of 20–25 cm H_2O; this is because in normal patients the lower esophageal tone is about 25 cm H_2O, and the risk to cause gastric insufflation and vomiting is lower.

The success of NPPV must be monitored with subjective and objective parameters. The early identification of NPPV failure is of pivotal importance for the outcome of the patient, <1 h. (Table 7.4)

7.4 Conclusion

Many studies comparing the Standard medical care (SMC) and the NPPV for ACPE and COPD show reduced hospital mortality and reduced endotracheal intubation rates and hospital length of stay.

In addition, there is little or no difference between NPPV and SCM for rate of acute myocardial infarction.

There aren't significant differences between patients with ACPE treated in the emergency room or intensive care unit.

It's important to provide guidelines in emergency department on when and how NPPV should be delivered.

Early treatment is of primary importance. Desirable for ACPE could be also start NPPV treatment out of hospital environment, appropriate selection of patients, skills of the attending staff are gold standard. Confirming the statement of Elliott et al.: "Staff training and experience is more important than location".

References

1. Lari F, Pilati G, Bragagni G, Di Battista N. Use of non-invasive ventilation for acute respiratory failure in general medical wards. Eur J Intern Med. 2008;19:S10–1.
2. Lightowler JV, Wedzicha JA, Elliott MW, et al. Non-invasive positive pressure ventilation to treat respiratory failure resulting from exacerbations of chronic obstructive pulmonary disease: Cochrane systematic review and meta-analysis. BMJ. 2003;326:185.
3. Meyer TJ. Hill ns, non-invasive positive pressure ventilation to treat respiratory failure. Ann Intern Med. 1994;120:760–70.
4. Dottorini M, Baglioni S, Eslami A, et al. N-CPAP in patients with COPD in acute respiratory failure. Chest. 1995;107:585–7.
5. Jeffery AA, Warren PM, Flenley DC. Acute hypercapnic respiratory failure in patients with chronic obstructive lung disease; risk factors and use of guidelines for management. Thorax. 1992;47:34–40.
6. Siafakas NM, Vermeire P, Pride NB, et al. Optimal assessment and management of chronic obstructive pulmonary disease (COPD). Eur Respir J. 1995;8:1398–420.
7. Rochwerg B, Brochard L, Elliott MW, et al. Official ERS/ATS clinical practice guidelines: non-invasive ventilation for acute respiratory failure. Eur Respir J. 2017;50:1602426.
8. Nava S, Hill N. Non-invasive ventilation in acute respiratory failure. Lancet. 2009;374:250–9.
9. Metha S, Jay GD, Woolard RH, et al. Randomized, prospective trial of bilevel versus continuous positive airway pressure in acute pulmonary edema. Crit Care Med. 1997;25:620–8.
10. Metha S, Al-Hashim AH, Keenan SP. Non-invasive ventilation in patient with acute cardiogenic pulmonary edema. Respir Care. 2009;54:186–95.

11. Gray A, Goodacre S, Newby DE, et al. Non-invasive ventilation in acute cardiogenic pulmonary edema. N Engl J Med. 2008;359:142–51.
12. Vital FM, Laidera MT, Atallah AN. Non-invasive positive pressure ventilation (CPA or bilevel NPPV) for cardiogenetic pulmonary oedema. Cochrane Database Syst Rev. 2013;5:CD005351.
13. Keenan SP, Sinuff BKE, et al. Canadian critical care trials group/Canadian critical care society non-invasive ventilation guidelines group. CMAJ. 2011;183:E195–214.
14. Mebazaa A, Yilmaz MB, Levy P, et al. Recommendations on prehospital and early hospital management of acute heart failure: a consensus paper from the heart failure Association of the European Society of Cardiology, the European Society of emergency medicine. Eur Heart J. 2015;36:1958–66.
15. Sanchez D, Smith G, Piper A, Roll K. Non-invasive ventilation guidelines for adult patient with acute failure: a clinical practice guideline. Agency for clinical Innovation NSW government Chatswood NSW; 2014.
16. Yancy W, Jessup M, Bozkurt B, et al. Guideline for the management of heart failure a report of the American College of Cardiology Foundation/American Heart Association ACCF/AHA 2013. Circulation. 2013;128(16):1810–52. https://doi.org/10.1161/CIR.0b013e31829e8807.
17. Vital PMR, Laidera MT, Atallah AN. Non-invasive positive pressure ventilation (CPAP or bilevel NPPV) for cardiogenic pulmonary oedema. Cochrane Database Syst Rev. 2013;5:CD005351.
18. Kallet RH, Diaz JV. The phisiologic effects of non-invasive ventilation. Respir Care. 2009;54:102–15.
19. Antonelli M, Conti G, Moro ML, et al. Predictor of failure of non-invasive positive pressure ventilation in patients with acute hypoxemic respiratory failure: a multicenter study. Intensive Care Med. 2001;27:1718–28.
20. Longhini F, Colombo D, Pisani L, Antonelli M, et al. Efficacy of ventilator waveform observation for detection of patient-ventilator asynchrony during NIV: a multicenter study. ERJ Open Res. 2017;3(4):00075–2017. https://doi.org/10.1183/23120541.00075-2017.

Critical Care Applications of NIMV and Related Issues: Critical Care

Non-invasive Positive Airway Pressure and Non-invasive Ventilation in Acute Cardiogenic Pulmonary Edema

8

Antonio Coviello, Ludovica Golino, and Ezio Spasari

Contents

Acute Cardiogenic Pulmonary Edema (ACPE) is a medical emergency that every year observes up to 1 million hospital admissions in the United States [1]. 6.5 million of hospitalization days are registered each year [2]. Hospital mortality from ACPE, especially when it is associated with acute myocardial infarction, is from 10% to 20% [3]. The prevalence of ACPE was estimated to be 75,000–83,000 cases per 100,000 individuals among heart failure patients with reduced ejection fraction. ACPE generally affects individuals older than 65 years where males are more commonly involved than females [4]. Patients who do not respond to medical therapy often require tracheal intubation and ventilation; in these cases there are more complication risks [5]. Tracheal intubation can be averted with the use of ventilation non-invasive methods by improving oxygenation, reducing the work of breathing, and increasing cardiac output [6–9].

A. Coviello (✉) · E. Spasari
Department of Neurosciences, Reproductive and Odontostomatological Sciences, University of Naples "Federico II", Naples, Italy

L. Golino
Anesthesia and Intensive Unit of Emergency Department, San Giovanni di Dio Hospital, Frattamaggiore, Italy

8.1   Acute Cardiogenic Pulmonary Edema

ACPE is a medical emergency which requires an immediate management. Lung fluid accumulation impairs gas exchange and lung compliance causing dyspnea and hypoxia [10]. All factors which contribute both to increased pressure and blood pooling on the heart left side can cause ACPE [11]. As a result, there will be an increase of: heart left side pressure; pulmonary venous pressure; lung capillary pressure.

ACPE produces a non-inflammatory edema due to Starling forces alteration. The normal range of pulmonary capillary pressures is from 6 to 13 mmHg, but any factor which increases these pressures can cause pulmonary edema [12]. Normally negative pressure in extra-alveolar interstitial spaces keeps dry alveoli, but when there is an increase of heart left side pressure, pulmonary venous pressure, lung capillary pressure induces fluids in interstitial spaces and successively in alveoli (pulmonary edema) [13].

ACPE causes can be: coronary artery diseases with left ventricular failure (myocardial infarction); congestive heart failure; cardiomyopathy; heart left side valvular diseases (stenosis and regurgitation); cardiac arrhythmias; right to left shunts.

A patient afflicted with ACPE shows pale, cool to touch and sweaty, breathless, and in upright sitting. Coughing up pink frothy sputum is relatively uncommon. Patients may have a central or peripheral cyanosis and reduced oxygen saturations.

A sensitive and specific diagnostic approach for ACPE is a critical issue. Accurate and rapid nature determination of acute dyspnea is an important and challenging matter in the Intensive Care Unit (ICU) and the Emergency Department (ED) [14]. The common diagnostic methods that are used to determine the cause of acute dyspnea include B-type Natriuretic Peptide (BNP) test, N-Terminal (NT) proBNP test, X-ray, ultrasound, and thoracic Computed Tomography (CT) scan.

ACPE often responds rapidly to medical treatment. Upright position may relieve symptoms. A loop diuretic such as furosemide is administered, often together with morphine to reduce respiratory distress. Both diuretic and morphine may have vasodilator effects, but specific vasodilators may be used (particularly nitroglycerin) if blood pressure is adequate, otherwise inotropes are needed in order to support blood circulation [15].

Supplemental oxygen therapy should be early started to treat hypoxemia ($SpO_2 < 90\%$) in such conditions. Venturi masks, reservoir masks, or nasal cannulas are widely used; however, Acute Respiratory Failure (ARF) is not often fully compensated with conventional oxygen treatment and may require greater respiratory support in order to achieve the target of an SpO_2 90–96%. Lower O_2 saturation target (88–92%) is recommended in patients with both acute heart failure and Chronic Obstructive Pulmonary Disease (COPD) [16].

Guidelines [17–21] demonstrated that Continuous Positive Airway Pressure (CPAP) and bilevel Non-Invasive Ventilation (NIV) reduce mortality and the need of invasive mechanical ventilation in people with severe cardiogenic pulmonary edema [22].

8.2   NIV and CPAP in ACPE: Pathophysiology and Benefit of Positive Airway Pressure

NIV makes use of mechanical respiratory support by techniques that do not bypass the upper airway. Nowadays, NIV is the recommended first-line method of ventilator support in selected patients with ARF of various origins, including ACPE, that is the most common cause of ARF [23].

NIV is generally practiced by using a combination of Pressure Support Ventilation (PSV) plus Positive End-Expiratory Pressure (PEEP), or Inspiratory Positive Airway Pressure (IPAP) with Expiratory Positive Airway Pressure (EPAP), obtaining a BiLevel (BiPAP) ventilation. Unlike NIV, CPAP is not considered a ventilation method because it does not support the inspiration phase and the ventilator does not cycle.

An extravascular lung water increase, a lung volumes and respiratory system compliance reduction, and an airway resistance increase are at the base of pathophysiology of ACPE [24]. Therefore, the consequences of these changes are an increased work of breathing and oxygen cost of breathing, with an imbalance between oxygen consumption and oxygen delivery [25, 26]. As to effects on hemodynamics during non-invasive airway pressure in patients with left heart failure, CPAP may reduce Left Ventricular (LV) afterload without compromising cardiac index [27, 28]. This is aided by the decreased negative pressure swings produced by the respiratory system. Furthermore, in patients presenting ACPE caused by a diastolic dysfunction, the hemodynamic benefit of CPAP is due to a decrease in LV end-diastolic volume (preload) following a reduced venous return [29].

There is considerable evidence that positive airway pressure reduces cardiac output by decreasing venous return [29–32].

Total venous return depends on a driving pressure gradient and the resistance to venous return. According to Guyton's theory, [33–35] the driving force is the difference between mean systemic filling pressure (Pms) and right atrial pressure (Pra).

For several years, it has been suggested that positive airway pressure, by increasing Pra, reduces venous return by decreasing the pressure gradient between Pms and Pra [36, 37]. However, experimental [38] and human [39] studies reported that positive airway pressure equally increased Pra and Pms and altered venous return with no impact on the pressure gradient (Pms − Pra). Accordingly, a decrease in blood flow resulting from the use of positive airway pressure was ascribed to an increased resistance to venous return. This concept was supported by experimental results [40] which suggested that application of PEEP would decrease blood flow not only by an increase in the liver venous back pressure to flow, but also by an increase in venous resistance caused by a compression of the liver by the diaphragm.

8.3 NIV vs CPAP in ACPE: Evidence-Based Results

In 2008, the largest randomized multicenter trial on the use of NIV in patients with ARF due to ACPE was published [41]. One thousand and sixty-nine patients belonging to 26 emergency departments in the United Kingdom were included in the study to receive standard oxygen therapy, CPAP (5–15 cm H2O), or NIV (inspiratory pressure, 8–20 cm H2O; expiratory pressure, 4–10 cm H2O).

Non-invasive ventilatory support delivered by either CPAP or NIV showed earlier improvement of dyspnea, respiratory distress, and metabolic alterations despite conventional oxygen therapy, although rates of survival did not improve [42]. Lately, five systematic reviews [43–46] concluded that NIV decreases the need for intubation and hospital mortality, and that NIV and CPAP have similar effects on the main outcomes.

In addition, a greater risk of myocardial infarction with NIV than with CPAP was detected in an early trial [47]. The latest European guidelines confirm the therapeutic equivalence of NIV and CPAP in ACPE. In conclusion, NIV or CPAP should be considered as a first-line strategy in the management of patients with ACPE because they decrease the need for Endotracheal Intubation (EI) and hospital mortality. Both techniques decrease the systemic venous return and the LV afterload, thus reducing LV filling pressure and limiting pulmonary edema. In the management of ACPE patients, CPAP and NIV have shown similar effects on the main outcomes, for this reason they may be used interchangeably. NIV has the potential advantage over CPAP of assisting the patient during inspiration, with relief of dyspnea and improvement of vital signs [47]. However, these physiological benefits were not translated into primary outcomes in clinical studies, which did not report significant differences between CPAP and NIV in terms of EI or survival [23]. CPAP might be considered first choice intervention, because of its easy use, cheap, and simple setting-up. The choice of one technique rather than another may depend on the type of patient, personal experience, treatment setting, etiology, and pathophysiology of the respiratory failure.

8.4 NIV and CPAP: Modes and Devices

As already mentioned, NIV is generally delivered by using an assisted ventilation with combination of PSV and PEEP or in BiPAP mode. NIV can be set also in Assist/Control (A/C) mode, in which the machine provides a tidal volume either when triggered by the patient (assist) or when the patient's inspiratory effort does not occur within a given period (control). In A/C ventilation, volume-cycled and pressure-targeted modes are available. Finally, in Neurally Adjusted Ventilatory Assist (NAVA), the ventilator adjusts mechanical assistance to the Electrical Activity of the diaphragm (EAdi), which can estimate the respiratory drive and trigger on and cycle off the delivery of ventilator assistance [48].

Unlike NIV, CPAP does not deliver ventilation because it does not assist inspiration and the ventilator does not cycle, but it rather delivers a constant pressure throughout the entire respiratory cycles. For spontaneous breathing that is not supported, this technique requires effective respiratory drive and maintained alveolar ventilation. As to ventilatory setting, low positive pressure should be initially delivered to enhance patient's tolerance (appropriate initial pressures are with CPAP 3–5 cm H2O and inspiratory pressure 8–12 cm H2O above CPAP). Pressure can be gradually increased, till tolerated, to deliver adequate tidal volumes, between 6 mL/kg and 8 mL/kg. The purpose is to relieve dyspnea, to reduce respiratory rate, and to ensure good patient-ventilator interaction.

Commonly, hypoxemic ARF patients receive CPAP levels in a range from 5 to 12 cm H2O and oxygen supplementation is titrated to an oxygen saturation target between 92% and 98%, or between 88% and 92% in patients at risk of hypercapnia (i.e., exacerbation of chronic respiratory failure).

Interfaces for NIV enable sealed connection between the ventilator circuit and the patients' airways, allowing delivery of pressure/flow into the lung. The choice of the suitable interface is among the most relevant issues to ensure NIV success. Alternating available interfaces may represent an effective approach to optimize comfort and tolerance, especially in patients undergoing prolonged treatments.

Available devices are: nasal mask, oro-nasal mask, full-face mask, and helmet; all these interfaces can be used with intensive care ventilators and bilevel ventilators.

CPAP can be applied by NIV devices with bilevel or intensive care ventilators, but also with various devices defined low gas flow generators with reservoir, high-flow jet venturi circuits, and high-flow nasal cannula. These levels are proportional to gas flow and are enhanced during preferential nose breathing [49, 50].

8.5 Clinical Management

CPAP or NIV trial should be considered in patients with respiratory distress, gas exchange abnormalities, accessory muscles use, and/or paradoxical abdominal breathing persistent on conventional oxygen therapy. However, the trial can be performed if emergent intubation is not indicated and no contraindications to NIV exist (Table 8.1).

When NIV trial is recommended, it should be initiated as soon as possible since delays could

Table 8.1 Contraindications for NIV

Absolute	• Need for emergent intubation
	• Respiratory arrest
	• Inability to protect the airway
	• Severe altered mental status
	• Shock/severe hemodynamic instability
	• Undrained pneumothorax
	• Bowel obstruction
Relative	• Nausea and vomiting
	• Copious secretions
	• Mild agitation/ uncooperative patients
	• Reduced consciousness
	• Facial, esophageal, or gastric surgery, trauma, burns, or deformity
	• Mild hypotension

Table 8.2 Risk factors of NIV failure

Prior to NIV	Hypotension with vasoprassor need Multiple organ failure Delayed onset Copious secretions Severe hypoxaemia Extremely high respiratory rate
After NIV initiation	Air leakage (inappropriate interface, intolerance to interface/agitation) Asynchrony with the ventilator/ inappropriate ventilator settings Respiratory rate > 30/min Low PH or high arterial carbon dioxide concentration No oxygenation improvement ($\downarrow SpO_2$ or $\downarrow PaO_2/FiO_2$)

result in worsening of clinical condition and NIV failure [51–53].

NIV is typically initiated in the hospital setting, but many studies suggest that prehospital CPAP or NIV administered by emergency medical transport personnel may reduce mortality and/or rates of intubation [54–61].

The success of the technique depends on both the underlying patient's condition and clinician and staff's expertise, patient's comfort, and tolerance during NIV trials. In this context, it is crucial to select the correct patients and interfaces in order to achieve a good synchrony between patients and the ventilator and minimize the failure risk (Table 8.2).

8.6 Modalities Selection and Settings

CPAP, BiPAP, and more recently, High Flow Nasal Cannula (HFNC) are the most common modes used.

Some authors suggest to initially deliver low pressures to enhance patient's tolerance and, if necessary, they can be gradually increased to reach adequate tidal volumes.

Some others suggest to deliver the highest tolerate pressures in order to quickly improve muscle fatigue, relieve dyspnea, and reduce respiratory rate. The lack of strong evidence supporting a technique rather than another could derive from the presence of a wide range of patient subgroups which differ for gravity, underlying conditions, and comorbidity.

General initial settings could be the following:

(a) *HFNC*: it could replace conventional O2 therapy in selected subgroups of patients. It is often started with FiO2 of 100% and flow levels as high as tolerated, then it should be decreased evaluating blood gas samples and clinical parameters.

(b) *CPAP*: it could be applied without the aid of a ventilator, by using a high flow source of air and/or oxygen to deliver gasses applying positive pressure (PEEP), using a Venturi tube, or the Boussignac system [62, 63]. CPAP is more indicated in areas not equipped with ventilators, but NIV is an appropriate alternative, especially when hypercapnia is present or if CPAP fails. CPAP could be initially set from 5 to 8 cm H2O and titrated up to 20 cm H2O according to the tolerance to achieve improvement of dyspnea and decreased respiratory rate.

(c) *BiPAP:* it is particularly helpful in patients with acute hypercapnic respiratory failure (COPD) and disorders associated with pump failure (drug overdose, neuromuscular disorders, or obesity). Bilevel NIV mode is often used in spontaneous/timed (S/T) setting with a backup rate from 8 breaths/ min to 12 breaths/min. The S/T setting is more often selected since it ensures that all breaths are supported and that a minimum respiratory rate is provided if the patient hyperventilates for whatever reason. In this context, IPAP could be set from 8 to 12 cm H2O. IPAP may be titrated upward according to the tolerance, usually incrementing of 2 cm H2O, to a maximum of 20 cm H2O. An adequate pressure should guarantee proportional tidal volume decreasing the work of breathing, improving ventilation, and minimizing asynchronies. EPAP could be set from 3 to 5 cm H2O, increasing (up to 10 cm H2O) to get better oxygenation. However, this maneuver may decrease the delivered tidal volume.

Fraction of inspired oxygen (FiO₂) as needed to keep peripheral O₂ saturation (SpO₂) > 90% considering the underlying disorder. Oxygen should be carefully administered as it may cause vasoconstriction and reduction in cardiac output [64].

8.7 Monitoring and Follow-Up

The treatment of ARF due to cardiogenic pulmonary edema needs a close monitoring of several parameters directly linked to patient clinical status, to the ventilator performance, and to the patient-device coupling [65].

Clinicians should frequently monitor level of consciousness, respiratory rate, heart rate, blood pressure, and SpO2. Arterial blood samples should be analyzed within 30–45 min after the application of HFNC, CPAP, or NIV and repeated at least at 60 min and/or 90–120 min. In addition, they can be taken—when indicated—in order to evaluate partial pressure of oxygen (PaO2), partial pressure of carbon dioxide (PaCO2), partial pressure of oxygen to fraction of oxygen ratio (PaO2/FiO2), pH, and lactate levels. Moreover, continuous display visualization of pressure and flow waveforms would allow to reduce asynchrony and discomfort which are among the most important causes of CPAP-NIV failure [66–68].

Alarms should be set to promptly identify apnea or high respiratory rate, low/high minute ventilation and tidal volume, and low/high airway pressure [69]. CPAP or NIV is usually stopped when clinical features are improved or if there are signs of NIV failure, requiring endotracheal intubation. No special weaning is required after short-term use of non-invasive ventilation (usually 1–6 h) with FiO2 < 0.5 and low PEEP; conversely, a weaning period is often carried out after mild-long-term therapies by decreasing progressively FiO2 and positive pressure support.

Monitoring and follow-up can be performed also with the use of lung ultrasound. Lung imaging was traditionally considered off-limits for ultrasound techniques. It is due to the acoustic barrier of high-impedance air wall (Fig. 8.1).

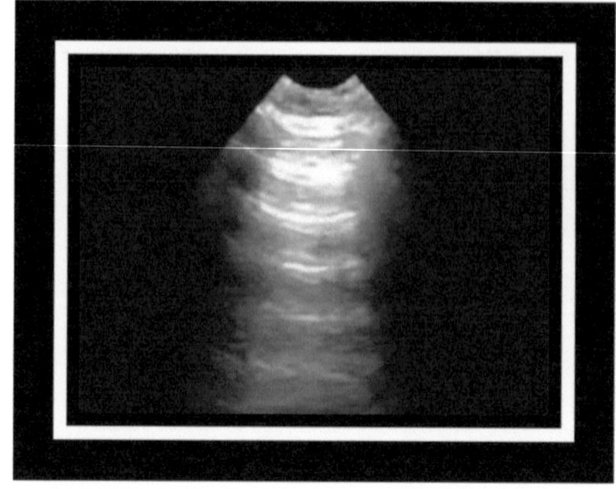

Fig. 8.1 A lines

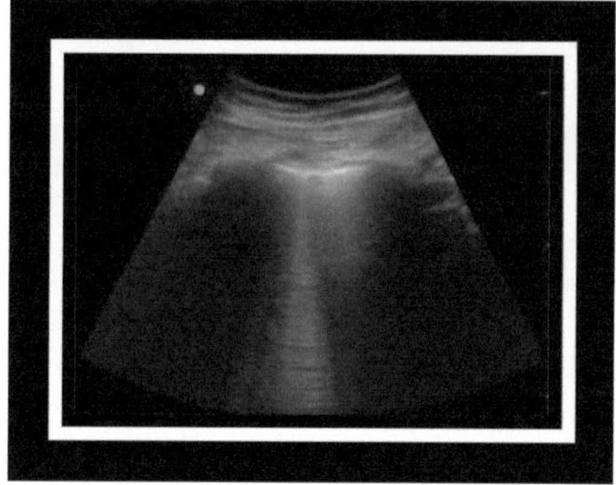

Fig. 8.2 B lines

Indeed, in pulmonary congestion, the presence of both air and water creates a peculiar echo fingerprint named B-lines (Fig. 8.2). Comet-like signals arise from a hyper-echoic pleural line with a to-and-fro movement synchronized with breathing [70]. The common lung image is modified from Extravascular Lung Water (EVLW) accumulation. In fact, the normal black lung pattern changes into a black-and-white pattern (interstitial subpleural edema with multiple B-lines) or into a white lung pattern (alveolar pulmonary edema) with coalescing B-lines [71]. B-lines represent 'the shape of lung water'. The number and spatial extent of B-lines allow a semiquantitative estimation of EVLW (from absent, ≤5, to severe pulmonary edema, >30 B-lines) (Fig. 8.3). B-lines can be evaluated anywhere, anytime, by

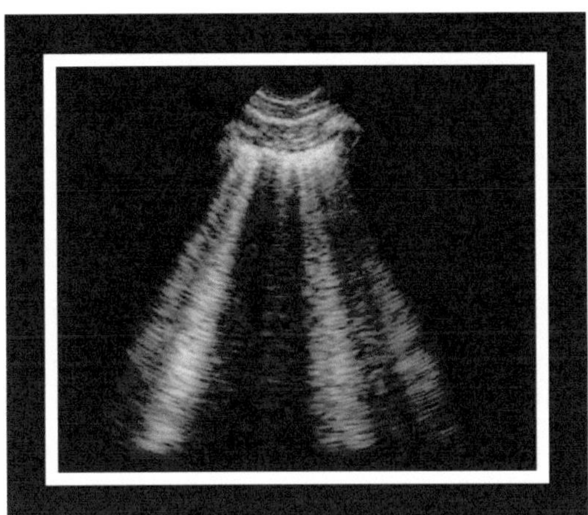

Fig. 8.3 Lung Rockets

anyone, and on anybody [72, 73]. They allow non-invasive and real time detection of even subclinical forms of pulmonary edema with a low cost and radiation-free approach.

8.8 Conclusions

HFNC, CPAP, or NIV are widely used in the treatment of ACPE, reducing the need of endotracheal intubation and the hospital mortality. These techniques should be used as a first-line therapy alongside conventional medical therapy. They can be adopted whenever patients with ACPE do not improve with standard oxygen therapy, if emergent intubation is not indicated, and no contraindication to NIV exists. Further research is needed to investigate whether NIV can be superior to CPAP in certain subgroups of patients. This study should include patients with coexisting respiratory disease such as COPD, valvular heart disease, low blood pressure, or with important muscle fatigue.

References

1. American Heart Association. Heart disease and stroke statistics—2005 update. Dallas: American Heart Association; 2005.
2. Felker GM, Adams KF Jr, Konstam MA, O'Connor CM, Gheorghiade M. The problem of decompensated heart failure: nomenclature, classification, and risk stratification. Am Heart J. 2003;145:S18–25.
3. Girou E, Brun-Buisson C, Taillé S, Lemaire F, Brochard L. Secular trends in nosocomial infections and mortality associated with noninvasive ventilation in patients with exacerbation of COPD and pulmonary edema. JAMA. 2003;290(22):2985–91.
4. Stevenson R, Ranjadayalan K, Wilkinson P, Roberts R, Timmis AD. Short and long term prognosis of acute myocardial infarction since introduction of thrombolysis. BMJ. 1993;307(6900):349–53.
5. British Thoracic Society Standards of Care Committee. Non-invasive ventilation in acute respiratory failure. Thorax. 2002;57(3):192–211.
6. Katz JA, Marks JD. Inspiratory work with and without continuous positive airway pressure in patients with acute respiratory failure. Anesthesiology. 1985;63(6):598–607.
7. Baratz DM, Westbrook PR, Shah PK, Mohsenifar Z. Effect of nasal continuous positive airway pressure on cardiac output and oxygen delivery in patients with congestive heart failure. Chest. 1992;102(5):1397–401.
8. Lenique F, Habis M, Lofaso F, DuboisRandé JL, Harf A, Brochard L. Ventilatory and hemodynamic effects of continuous positive airway pressure in left heart failure. Am J Respir Crit Care Med. 1997;155(2):500–5.
9. Naughton MT, Rahman MA, Hara K, Floras JS, Bradley TD. Effect of continuous positive airway pressure on intrathoracic and left ventricular transmural pressures in patients with congestive heart failure. Circulation. 1995;91(6):1725–31.
10. Powell J, Graham D, O'Reilly S, Punton G. Acute pulmonary oedema. Nurs Stand. 2016;30(23):51–9.
11. Sureka B, Bansal K, Arora A. Pulmonary edema-cardiogenic or noncardiogenic? J Family Med Prim Care. 2015;4(2):290.
12. Murray JF. Pulmonary edema: pathophysiology and diagnosis. Int J Tuberc Lung Dis. 2011;15(2):155–60.
13. Sibbald WJ, Anderson RR, Holliday RL. Pathogenesis of pulmonary edema associated with the adult respiratory distress syndrome. Can Med Assoc J. 1979;120(4):445–50.
14. Nielsen LS, Svanegaard J, Wiggers P, Egeblad H. The yield of a diagnostic hospital dyspnoea clinic for the primary health care section. J Intern Med. 2001;250(5):422–8.
15. Cleland JG, Yassin AS, Khadjooi K. Acute heart failure: focusing on acute cardiogenic pulmonary oedema. Clin Med. 2010;10(1):59–64.
16. O'Driscoll BR, Howard LS, Earis J, et al. BTS guideline for oxygen use in adults in healthcare and emergency settings. Thorax. 2017;72:ii1–ii90.
17. McMurray JJ, Adamopoulos S, Anker SD, Auricchio A, Böhm M, Dickstein K, Falk V, Filippatos G, Fonseca C, Gomez-Sanchez MA, Jaarsma T, Køber L, Lip GY, Maggioni AP, Parkhomenko A, Pieske BM, Popescu BA, Rønnevik PK, Rutten FH, Schwitter J, Seferovic P, Stepinska J, Trindade PT, Voors AA,

Zannad F, Zeiher A. ESC guidelines for the diagnosis and treatment of acute and chronic heart failure 2012: the task force for the diagnosis and treatment of acute and chronic heart failure 2012 of the European Society of Cardiology. Developed in collaboration with the heart failure association (HFA) of the ESC. Eur Heart J. 2012;33(14):1787–847.

18. National Clinical Guideline Centre (UK). Acute heart failure. Diagnosing and managing acute heart failure in adults, 2014;

19. Rochwerg B, Brochard L, Elliott MW, Hess D, Hill NS, Nava S, Navalesi P, Antonelli M, Brozek J, Conti G, Ferrer M, Guntupalli K, Jaber S, Keenan S, Mancebo J, Mehta S, Raoof S. Official ERS/ATS clinical practice guidelines: noninvasive ventilation for acute respiratory failure. Eur Respir J. 2017;50(2):1602426.

20. Chawla R, Dixit SB, Zirpe KG, Chaudhry D, Khilnani GC, Mehta Y, Khatib KI, Jagiasi BG, Chanchalani G, Mishra RC, Samavedam S, Govil D, Gupta S, Prayag S, Ramasubban S, Dobariya J, Marwah V, Sehgal I, Jog SA, Kulkarni AP. ISCCM guidelines for the use of non-invasive ventilation in acute respiratory failure in adult ICUs. Indian J Crit Care Med. 2020;24:61–81.

21. Akashiba T, Ishikawa Y, Ishihara H, Imanaka H, Ohi M, Ochiai R, Kasai T, Kimura K, Kondoh Y, Sakurai S, Shime N, Suzukawa M, Takegami M, Takeda S, Tasaka S, Taniguchi H, Chohnabayashi N, Chin K, Tsuboi T, Tomii K, Narui K, Hasegawa N, Hasegawa R, Ujike Y, Kubo K, Hasegawa Y, Momomura SI, Yamada Y, Yoshida M, Takekawa Y, Tachikawa R, Hamada S, Murase K. The Japanese respiratory society noninvasive positive pressure ventilation (NPPV) guidelines (second revised edition). Respir Investig. 2017;55(1):83–92.

22. Wang Y, Brown J, Godfrey C, Ahmad M, Vital FMR, Lambiase P, Banerjee A, Bakhai A, Chong M. Non-invasive positive pressure ventilation (CPAP or bilevel NPPV) for cardiogenic pulmonary oedema. Cochrane Database Syst Rev. 2019;4(4):CD005351.

23. Rochwerg B, Brochard L, Elliott MW, et al. Official ERS/ATS clinical practice guidelines: noninvasive ventilation for acute respiratory failure. Eur Respir J. 2017;50(2):1602426.

24. Sharp JT, Griffith GT, Bunnell IL, et al. Ventilatory mechanics in pulmonary edema in man. J Clin Invest. 1958;37(1):111–7.

25. Aubier M, Trippenbach T, Roussos C. Respiratory muscle fatigue during cardiogenic shock. J Appl Physiol. 1981;51(2):499–508.

26. Field S, Kelly SM, Macklem PT. The oxygen cost of breathing in patients with cardiorespiratory disease. Am Rev Respir Dis. 1982;126(1):9–13.

27. Räsänen J, Heikkilä J, Downs J, et al. Continuous positive airway pressure by face mask in acute cardiogenic pulmonary edema. Am J Cardiol. 1985;325(26):1825–30.

28. Naughton MT, Rahman MA, Hara K, et al. Effect of continuous positive airway pressure on intrathoracic and left ventricular transmural pressures in patients with congestive heart failure. Circulation. 1995;91(6):1725–31.

29. Bendjelid K, Schütz N, Suter PM, et al. Does continuous positive airway pressure by face mask improve patients with acute cardiogenic pulmonary edema due to left ventricular diastolic dysfunction? Chest. 2005;127(3):1053–8.

30. Dhainaut JF, Devaux JY, Monsallier JF, et al. Mechanisms of decreased left ventricular preload during continuous positive pressure ventilation in ARDS. Chest. 1986;90(1):74–80.

31. Schuster S, Erbel R, Weilemann LS, et al. Hemodynamics during PEEP ventilation in patients with severe left ventricular failure studied by transesophageal echocardiography. Chest. 1990;97(5):1181–9.

32. Leithner C, Podolsky A, Globits S, et al. Magnetic resonance imaging of the heart during positive end-expiratory pressure ventilation in normal subjects. Crit Care Med. 1994;22(3):426–32.

33. Guyton AC. Determination of cardiac output by equating venous return curves with cardiac response curves. Physiol Rev. 1955;35(1):123–9.

34. Guyton AC, Lindsey AW, Abernathy B, et al. Venous return at various right atrial pressures and the normal venous return curve. Am J Phys. 1957;189(3):609–15.

35. Magder S. Volume and its relationship to cardiac output and venous return. Crit Care. 2016;20(1):271.

36. Cournand A, Motley HL, Werkio L, et al. Physiological studies of the effects of intermittent positive pressure breathing on cardiac output in man. Am J Phys. 1948;152(1):162–74.

37. Braunwald E, Binion JT, Morgan WL, et al. Alterations in central blood volume and cardiac output induced by positive pressure breathing counteracted by metaraminol (Aramine). Circ Res. 1957;5(6):670–5.

38. Fessler HE, Brower RG, Wise RA, et al. Effects of positive end-expiratory pressure on the gradient for venous return. Am Rev Respir Dis. 1991;143(1):19–24.

39. Nanas S, Magder S. Adaptations of the peripheral circulation to PEEP. Am Rev Respir Dis. 1992;146(3):688–93.

40. Brienza N, Revelly JP, Ayuse T, et al. Effects of PEEP on liver arterial and venous blood flows. Am J Respir Crit Care Med. 1995;152(2):504–10.

41. Gray A, Goodacre S, Newby DE, et al. Noninvasive ventilation in acute cardiogenic pulmonary edema. N Engl J Med. 2008;359(2):142–51.

42. Potts JM. Noninvasive positive pressure ventilation: effect on mortality in acute cardiogenic pulmonary edema: a pragmatic meta-analysis. Pol Arch Med Wewn. 2009;119(6):349–53.

43. Weng CL, Zhao YT, Liu QH, et al. Meta-analysis: noninvasive ventilation in acute cardiogenic pulmonary edema. Ann Intern Med. 2010;152(9):590–600.

44. Mariani J, Macchia A, Belziti C, et al. Noninvasive ventilation in acute cardiogenic pulmonary edema: a meta-analysis of randomized controlled trials. J Card Fail. 2011;17(10):850–9.

45. Vital FM, Ladeira MT, Atallah AN. Non-invasive positive pressure ventilation (CPAP or bilevel NPPV) for cardiogenic pulmonary oedema. Cochrane Database Syst Rev. 2013;5:CD005351.
46. Cabrini L, Landoni G, Oriani A, et al. Noninvasive ventilation and survival in acute care settings: a comprehensive systematic review and metaanalysis of randomized controlled trials. Crit Care Med. 2015;43(4):880–8.
47. Mehta S, Jay GD, Woolard RH, et al. Randomized, prospective trial of bilevel versus continuous positive airway pressure in acute pulmonary edema. Crit Care Med. 1997;25(4):620–8.
48. Sinderby C, Navalesi P, Beck J, et al. Neural control of mechanical ventilation in respiratory failure. Nat Med. 1999;5(12):1433–6.
49. Parke RL, McGuinness SP. Pressures delivered by nasal high flow oxygen during all phases of the respiratory cycle. Respir Care. 2013;58(10):1621–4.
50. Chanques G, Riboulet F, Molinari N, et al. Comparison of three high flow oxygen therapy delivery devices: a clinical physiological cross-over study. Minerva Anestesiol. 2013;79(12):1344–55.
51. Nava S, Navalesi P, Conti G. Time of non-invasive ventilation. Intensive Care Med. 2006;32:361.
52. Collaborative Research Group of Noninvasive Mechanical Ventilation for Chronic Obstructive Pulmonary Disease. Early use of non-invasive positive pressure ventilation for acute exacerbations of chronic obstructive pulmonary disease: a multicentre randomized controlled trial. Chin Med J. 2005;118:2034.
53. Ozsancak Ugurlu A, Sidhom SS, Khodabandeh A, et al. Use and outcomes of noninvasive positive pressure ventilation in acute care hospitals in Massachusetts. Chest. 2014;145:964.
54. Thompson J, Petrie DA, Ackroyd-Stolarz S, Bardua DJ. Out-of-hospital continuous positive airway pressure ventilation versus usual care in acute respiratory failure: a randomized controlled trial. Ann Emerg Med. 2008;52:232.
55. Roessler MS, Schmid DS, Michels P, et al. Early out-of-hospital non-invasive ventilation is superior to standard medical treatment in patients with acute respiratory failure: a pilot study. Emerg Med J. 2012;29:409.
56. Plaisance P, Pirracchio R, Berton C, et al. A randomized study of out-of-hospital continuous positive airway pressure for acute cardiogenic pulmonary oedema: physiological and clinical effects. Eur Heart J. 2007;28:2895.
57. Goodacre S, Stevens JW, Pandor A, et al. Prehospital noninvasive ventilation for acute respiratory failure: systematic review, network meta-analysis, and individual patient data meta-analysis. Acad Emerg Med. 2014;21:960.
58. Bakke SA, Botker MT, Riddervold IS, et al. Continuous positive airway pressure and noninvasive ventilation in prehospital treatment of patients with acute respiratory failure: a systematic review of controlled studies. Scand J Trauma Resusc Emerg Med. 2014;22:69.
59. Aguilar SA, Lee J, Dunford JV, et al. Assessment of the addition of prehospital continuous positive airway pressure (CPAP) to an urban emergency medical services (EMS) system in persons with severe respiratory distress. J Emerg Med. 2013;45:210.
60. Mal S, McLeod S, Iansavichene A, et al. Effect of out-of-hospital noninvasive positive-pressure support ventilation in adult patients with severe respiratory distress: a systematic review and meta-analysis. Ann Emerg Med. 2014;63:600.
61. Ponikowski P, Voors AA, Anker SD, Bueno H, Cleland JG, Coats AJ, Falk V, González-Juanatey JR, Harjola VP, Jankowska EA, Jessup M, Linde C, Nihoyannopoulos P, Parissis JT, Pieske B, Riley JP, Rosano GM, Ruilope LM, Ruschitzka F, Rutten FH, van der Meer P. 2016 ESC guidelines for the diagnosis and treatment of acute and chronic heart failure. Eur Heart J. 2016;37(27):2129–200.
62. Brusasco C, Corradi F, De Ferrari A, Ball L, Kacmarek RM, Pelosi P. CPAP device for emergency prehospital use: a bench study. Respir Care. 2015;60(12):1777–85.
63. Vargas M, Marra A, Vivona L, Ball L, Marinò V, Pelosi P, Servillo G. Performances of CPAP devices with an oronasal mask. Respir Care. 2018;63(8):1033–9.
64. Park JH, Balmain S, Berry C, et al. Potentially detrimental cardiovascular effects of oxygen in patients with chronic left ventricular systolic dysfunction. Heart. 2010;96:553.
65. Rodríguez Mulero L, Carrillo Alcaraz A, Melgarejo Moreno A, Renedo Villarroya A, Párraga Ramírez M, Jara Pérez P, Millán MJ, González DG. Predictive factors related to success of noninvasive ventilation and mortality in the treatment of acute cardiogenic pulmonary edema. Med Clin (Barc). 2005;124(4):126–31.
66. Hess DR. Patent-ventilator interaction during noninvasive ventilation. Respir Care. 2011;56(2):153–65.
67. Thille A, Rodriguez P, Cabello B, Lellouche F, Brochard L. Patient-ventilator asynchrony during assisted mechanical ventilation. Intensive Care Med. 2006;32(10):1515–22.
68. Vignaux L, Vargas F, Roeseler J, Tassaux D, Thille AW, Kossowsky MP, Brochard L, Jolliet P. Patient-ventilator asynchrony during non-invasive ventilation for acute respiratory failure: a multicenter study. Intensive Care Med. 2009;35(5):840–6.
69. Di Marco F, Centanni S, Bellone A, Messinesi G, Pesci A, Scala R, Perren A. Nava S optimization of ventilator setting by flow and pressure waveforms analysis during noninvasive ventilation for acute exacerbations of COPD: a multicentric randomized controlled trial. Crit Care. 2011;15(6):R283.
70. Lichtenstein D, Me'zie're G, Biderman P, Gepner A, Barre´ O. The comet-tail artifact. An ultrasound sign of alveolar-interstitial syndrome. Am J Respir Crit Care Med. 1997;156(5):1640–6.
71. Jambrik Z, Monti S, Coppola V, Agricola E, Mottola G, Miniati M, Picano E. Usefulness of ultrasound

lung comets as a nonradiologic sign of extravascular lung water. Am J Cardiol. 2004;93(10):1265–70.

72. Picano E, Frassi F, Agricola E, Gligorova S, Gargani L, Mottola G. Ultrasound lung comets: a clinically useful sign of extravascular lung water. J Am Soc Echocardiogr. 2006;19(3):356–63.

73. Volpicelli G, Elbarbary M, Blaivas M, Lichtenstein DA, Mathis G, Kirkpatrick AW, Melniker L, Gargani L, Noble VE, Via G, Dean A, Tsung JW, Soldati G, Copetti R, Bouhemad B, Reissig A, Agricola E, Rouby JJ, Arbelot C, Liteplo A, Sargsyan A, Silva F, Hoppmann R, Breitkreutz R, Seibel A, Neri L, Storti E, Petrovic T. International liaison committee on lung ultrasound (ILC-LUS) for international consensus conference on lung ultrasound (ICC-LUS). International evidence-based recommendations for point-of-care lung ultrasound. Intensive Care Med. 2012;38(4):577–91.

Non-invasive Ventilation in Severe Pneumonia

9

Giuseppe Servillo, Pasquale Buonanno,
Andrea Uriel de Siena, Raffaele Merola,
and Ivana Capuano

Contents

9.1   Introduction

NIV is widely used in the acute care setting for acute respiratory failure (ARF) across a variety of etiologies [1]. NIV has become the first-choice ventilation technique in many clinical conditions, such as acute hypercapnic respiratory failure secondary to chronic obstructive pulmonary disease (COPD) and cardiogenic pulmonary edema, severe hypoxemia in immunosuppressed patients, and in order to facilitate the transition from invasive mechanical ventilation (IMV) to spontaneous breathing [2–4].

Less clear, however, is the role of NIV in patients with hypoxemic acute respiratory failure (HARF) due to pneumonia, acute respiratory distress syndrome (ARDS), and fibrosis.

In this chapter, we will focus only on the use of NIV in patients with severe acute respiratory failure (ARF) due to community-acquired pneumonia (CAP).

9.2   NIV in Severe Pneumonia

In recent years, the number of patients requiring intensive care management due to severe community-acquired pneumonia (SCAP) has globally increased, especially among the elderly, comorbid, and immunocompromised patients [5]. A recent study found that 21% of the patients hospitalized for CAP required an admission in intensive care unit (ICU), with 26% of them needing mechanical ventilation [6]. SCAP hospital mortality is still high, ranging from 25% to over 50% [7, 8]. The cornerstones of the pneumonia treatment are antibiotic therapy and ventilatory support in patients with ARF [9]. Invasive mechanical ventilation (IMV) implies numerous complications (e.g., ventilator-associated pneumonia, tracheal lesion and stenosis, respiratory muscle atrophy, ulceration, granulation tissue formation) [10, 11]. Therefore, NIV has been

G. Servillo · P. Buonanno (✉) · A. U. de Siena ·
R. Merola · I. Capuano
Department of Neurosciences and Reproductive and
Odontostomatological Sciences, University of Naples
"Federico II", Naples, Italy

G. Servillo, M. Vargas (eds.), *Non-invasive Mechanical Ventilation in Critical Care, Anesthesiology
and Palliative Care*, https://doi.org/10.1007/978-3-031-36510-2_9

used to avoid intubation and it showed satisfactory results in ARF of different etiology even if there is no definitive conclusions about the use of NIV in the treatment of SCAP [2–4].A Cochrane review including five RCTs found that NIV reduces the risk of hospital-acquired pneumonia in patient with COPD [12].

The efficacy of NIV in the course of pneumonia was investigated in a controlled trial of 56 patients randomized to receive either conventional treatment associated with NIV or conventional treatment alone [13]. The need for tracheal intubation was significantly lower in the group of patients treated with NIV (21% vs. 50%, $p < 0.03$), although the length of hospital stay and hospital mortality did not differ significantly. In a subgroup analysis, patients with COPD and hypercapnic respiratory failure enrolled in the NIV group had significantly lower 2-month mortality compared to the other group (11% vs. 63%, $p = 0.05$), while non-COPD patients treated with NIV did not show any advantage.

Jolliet et al. used face mask NIV in 24 patients with severe respiratory failure secondary to CAP; despite an initial improvement in oxygenation and a reduction in respiratory rate in almost all patients, the use of tracheal intubation was very high (66%) [14].

In a more recent prospective randomized trial in patients with HARF treated with NIV, the subgroup of patients with pneumonia had a reduced need for tracheal intubation and a reduction in mortality in ICU [15]. NIV was applied in 51 patients needing intubation for 24 h. This study suggests that NIV decreases the need for intubation, the incidence of septic shock, and the ICU mortality and increases the cumulative 90-day survival ($p = 0.025$), but arterial hypoxemia and tachypnea were higher in the non-invasive ventilation group treated with high-concentration oxygen therapy. Multivariate analyses showed NIV to be independently associated with decreased risks of intubation (odds ratio, 0.20; $p = 0.003$) and 90-day mortality (odds ratio, 0.39; $p = 0.017$).

In addition, pneumonia as the etiology of ARF is independently associated with the risk of NIV failing [16]. Patients with pneumonia share the same risk factors as other patients with HARF, but are also at risk of NIV failing if the infiltrates found on chest radiograph worsen in the 24 h after treatment with NIV [17]. Severity score at hospital admission (APACHE II, SAPSII, CURB65, Opravil Score), poor respiratory and cardiovascular function, the need for vasoactive drugs, organ dysfunction, worsening of Oxygenation Index in the first hour, and minute ventilation greater than 11 L/min at 48 h were independent risk factors for NIV failure [16–24] (Table 9.1).

Furthermore, delaying intubation in patients with pneumonia treated with NIV increases the risk of mortality in de novo respiratory failure [20]. The success of NIV therapy in patients with pneumonia who have not underlying acute-on-chronic respiratory failure requires careful attention to risk factors of failure and their management needs an experienced team of health-care providers [4].

According to these evidences, we can suggest a flowchart to decide when NIV is an effective alternative (Fig. 9.1).

Table 9.1 Predictor of NIV failure

Timing	Evaluation
Admission	APACHE IISAPS IICURB65higher LDHlower P/Fhigher A-aDO2older agehigher TV
Score after 1 h	P/F not improvinghigher TV
Score after 2 h	APACHE IIhigher TV
Score after 24 h	Opravil scoreSOFAhigher TV

TV tidal volume, *P/F* PaO_2/FiO_2, *LDH* lactate dehydrogenase

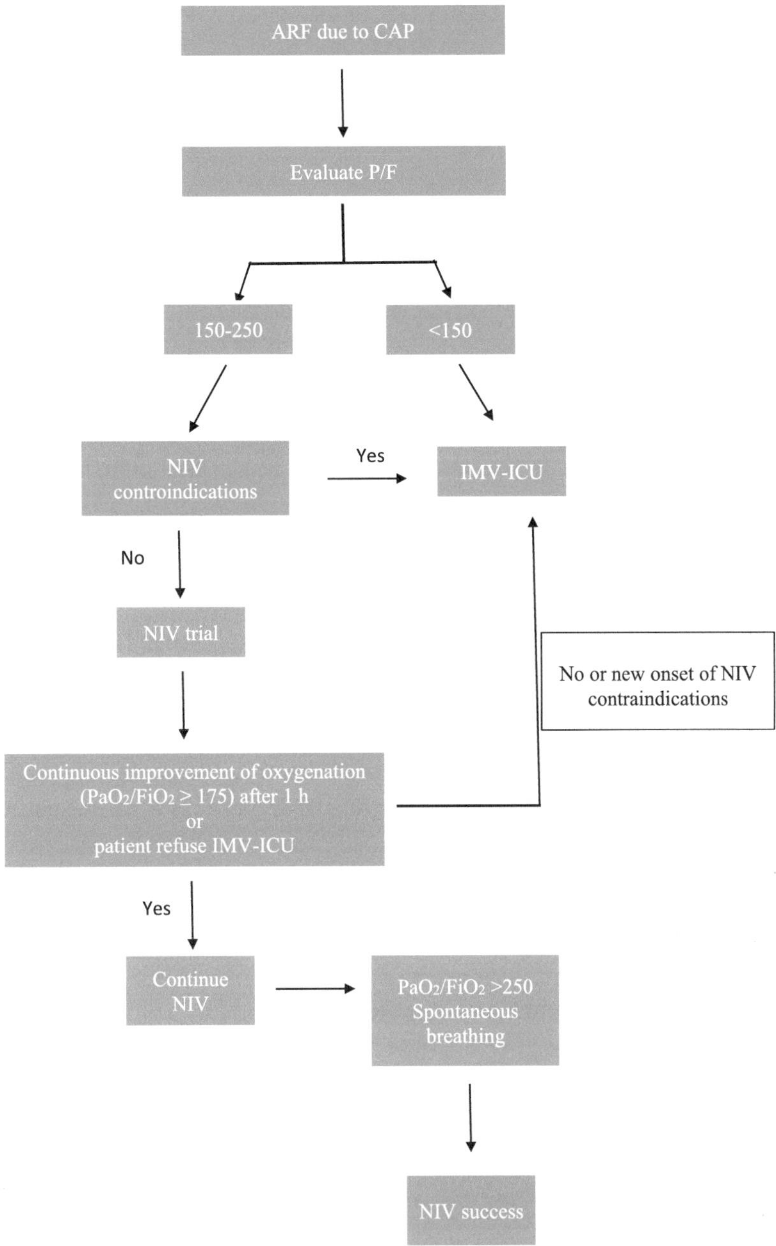

Fig. 9.1 Flowchart of NIV use in pneumonia

9.3 Conclusions

In conclusion, NIV can be an alternative to IMV in very selected patients suffering from severe pneumonia; pneumonia in COPD and hypercapnic patients seems to be the ideal condition in which NIV can be effective and avoid the need for tracheal intubation with all the consequences that IMV implies. For the patients suffering from severe pneumonia with a do not intubate order, NIV remains the only alternative to guarantee a ventilation support and it can be used as palliative measure. Furthermore, NIV can be the judgment call in the scenario of an unbalanced ratio between the available number of ICU beds and patients needing ICU admission as we experienced in COVID-19 pandemic: even in this situation NIV can be used for both therapeutic and palliative purposes.

References

1. Nava S, Hill N. Non-invasive ventilation in acute respiratory failure. Lancet. 2009;374:250–9.
2. Rochwerg B, Brochard L, Elliott MW, et al. Official ERS/ATS clinical practice guidelines: noninvasive ventilation for acute respiratory failure. Eur Respir J. 2017;50:1602426.
3. Pisani L, Corcione N, Nava S. Management of acute hypercapnic respiratory failure. Curr Opin Crit Care. 2016;22:45–52.
4. Brochard L, Lefebvre JC, Cordioli RL, et al. Noninvasive ventilation for patients with hypoxemic acute respiratory failure. Semin Respir Crit Care Med. 2014;35:492–500.
5. Laporte L, Hermetet C, Jouan Y, Gaborit C, Rouve E, Shea KM, Si-Tahar M, Dequin PF, Grammatico-Guillon L, Guillon A. Ten-year trends in intensive care admissions for respiratory infections in the elderly. Ann Intensive Care. 2018;8:84.
6. Jain S, Self WH, Wunderink RG, Fakhran S, Balk R, Bramley AM, Reed C, Grijalva CG, Anderson EJ, Courtney DM, Chappell JD, Qi C, Hart EM, Carroll F, Trabue C, Donnelly HK, Williams DJ, Zhu Y, Arnold SR, Ampofo K, Waterer GW, Levine M, Lindstrom S, Winchell JM, Katz JM, Erdman D, Schneider E, Hicks LA, McCullers JA, Pavia AT, Edwards KM, Finelli L. Community-acquired pneumonia requiring hospitalization among U.S. adults. N Engl J Med. 2015;373:415–27.
7. Cilloniz C, Dominedo C, Garcia-Vidal C, Torres A. Community-acquired pneumonia as an emergency condition. Curr Opin Crit Care. 2018;24:531–9.
8. Montull B, Menendez R, Torres A, Reyes S, Mendez R, Zalacain R, Cape-lastegui A, Rajas O, Borderias L, Martin-Villasclaras J, Bello S, Alfageme I, Rodriguez de Castro F, Rello J, Molinos L, Ruiz-Manzano J. Predictors of severe sepsis among patients hospitalized for community-acquired pneumonia. PLoS One. 2016;11:e0145929.
9. Pierson DJ. Indications for mechanical ventilation in adults with acute respiratory failure. Respir Care. 2002;47:249–62.
10. Chastre J, Fagon JY. Ventilator-associated pneumonia. Am J Respir Crit Care Med. 2002;165:867–903.
11. Slutsky AS, Ranieri VM. Ventilator-induced lung injury. N Engl J Med. 2013;369:2126–36.
12. Masterton RG, Galloway A, French G, Street M, Armstrong J, Brown E, Cleverley J, Dilworth P, Fry C, Gascoigne AD, Knox A, Nathwani D, Spencer R, Wilcox M. Guidelines for the management of hospital-acquired pneumonia in the UK: report of the working party on hospital-acquired pneumonia of the British society for antimicrobial chemotherapy. J Antimicrob Chemother. 2008;62(1):5–34. https://doi.org/10.1093/jac/dkn162.
13. Confalonieri M, Potena A, Carbone G, Della Porta R, Tolley E, Meduri G. Acute respiratory failure in patients with severe community-acquired pneumonia. A prospective randomized evaluation of noninvasive ventilation. Am J Respir Crit Care Med. 1999;160:1585–91.
14. Jolliet P, Abajo B, Pasquina P, Chevrolet JC. Non-invasive pressure support ventilation in severe community-acquired pneumonia. Intensive Care Med. 2001;27:812–21.
15. Ferrer M, Esquinas A, Leon M, Gonzalez G, Alarcon A, Torres A. Noninvasive ventilation in severe hypoxemic respiratory failure: a randomized clinical trial. Am J Respir Crit Care Med. 2003;168:1438–44.
16. Antonelli M, Conti G, Moro ML, Esquinas A, Gonzalez-Diaz G, Confalonieri M, et al. Predictors of failure of noninvasive positive pressure ventilation in patients with acute hypoxemic respiratory failure: a multi-center study. Intensive Care Med. 2001;27(11):1718–28.
17. Carrillo A, Gonzalez-Diaz G, Ferrer M, Martinez-Quintana ME, Lo-pez-Martinez A, Llamas N, et al. Non-invasive ventilation in community-acquired pneumonia and severe acute respiratory failure. Intensive Care Med. 2012;38(3):458–66.
18. Carron M, Freo U, Zorzi M, Ori C. Predictors of failure of noninvasive ventilation in patients with severe community-acquired pneumonia. J Crit Care. 2010;25:514–40.
19. Demoule A, Girou E, Richard JC, Taille S, Brochard L. Benefits and risks of success or failure of noninvasive ventilation. Intensive Care Med. 2006;32:1756–65.
20. Bellani G, Laffey JG, Pham T, Madotto F, Fan E, Brochard L, et al. LUNG SAFE investigators, ESICM trials group. Noninvasive ven-tilation of patients with acute respiratory distress syndrome. Insights from the LUNG SAFE study. Am J Respir Crit Care Med. 2017;195(1):67–77.
21. Murad A, Li PZ, Dial S, Shahin J. The role of non-invasive positive pressure ventilation in community-acquired pneumonia. J Crit Care. 2015;30(1):49–54.
22. Trivedi TH. Relying on radiological findings in critically ill H1N1 infected patients-how logical. J Assoc Physicians India. 2013;61:9–10.
23. He H, Sun B, Liang L, Li Y, Wang H, Wei L, et al. A multicenter RCT of noninvasive ventilation in pneumonia-induced early mild acute respiratory distress syndrome. Crit Care. 2019;23(1):300.
24. Nicolini A, Cilloniz C, Piroddi IM, Faverio P. Noninvasive ventilation for acute respiratory failure due to community-acquired pneumonia: a concise review and update. Community Acquired Infection. 2015;2(2):46–50.

Non-invasive Ventilation in Acute and Chronic Obstructive Pulmonary Disease

10

G. Castellano, A. Marra, L. Palumbo,
M. Melchionna, and Giuseppe Servillo

Contents

Respiratory failure from acute exacerbations of chronic obstructive pulmonary disease (COPD) or severe asthma is characterized by acute worsening of respiratory symptoms associated with the development of severe airflow limitation, gas trapping, dynamic hyperinflation, and intrinsic positive end-expiratory pressure (PEEPi). In the most severe cases, these exacerbations may cause acute respiratory failure, which may require mechanical ventilation [1].

COPD exacerbations are common and have important clinical consequences, including an acute decline in quality of life, temporary or permanent reduction in lung function and exercise capacity, hospitalization, and increased mortality, and major economic impact. According to cohort studies, the rate of non-invasive ventilation (NIV) as first ventilatory support in intensive care unit (ICU) in COPD patients increased from 16% in 1998 to 51% in 2017. Simultaneously, overall mortality decreased.

Severe asthma exacerbation causing respiratory failure may lead to major mechanical ventilation-associated complications (e.g., barotrauma, cardiovascular collapse, atelectasis, and pneumonia) that can impact morbidity and mortality. Severe asthma exacerbation accounts for approximately 1% of mechanically ventilated patients admitted to the ICU [2] and NIV use in these patients increased from 3% in 1998 to 34% in 2016 [3].

G. Castellano (✉) · L. Palumbo
Department of Anesthesia and Intensive Care,
Gemelli Molise Hospital, Campobasso, Italy

A. Marra · G. Servillo
Department of Neurosciences, Reproductive and
Odontostomatological Sciences, University of Naples
"Federico II", Naples, Italy

M. Melchionna
Clinical Pharmacy Gemelli Molise Hospital,
Campobasso, Italy

© The Author(s), under exclusive license to Springer Nature Switzerland AG 2023
G. Servillo, M. Vargas (eds.), *Non-invasive Mechanical Ventilation in Critical Care, Anesthesiology
and Palliative Care*, https://doi.org/10.1007/978-3-031-36510-2_10

10.1 Respiratory System Mechanics and Gas Exchange

In terms of respiratory system mechanics, COPD and asthma are characterized by the development of dynamic hyperinflation, defined as increased relaxation volume of the respiratory system at the end of a tidal expiration. In healthy subjects, the end expiratory alveolar and airway pressures are zero relative to the atmosphere, and pleural pressure is negative. In the presence of dynamic hyperinflation, the alveolar pressure remains positive throughout expiration, leading to the development of auto-positive end-expiratory pressure (auto-PEEP), also termed intrinsic PEEP or PEEPi [4].

In COPD, PEEPi is primarily caused by expiratory flow limitation, due to reduced lung recoil pressure leading to small airway collapse that increases airway resistance [5]. It is exacerbated by shortened expiratory time, due to increased respiratory rate, and increased tidal volume, the latter being, in general, a consequence of an augmentation of respiratory drive (and therefore a higher volume to exhale) [6]. In passively ventilated patients, dynamic hyperinflation increases delivered mechanical power [7] with its associated risk of barotrauma and hemodynamic compromise [8]. In patients triggering their ventilator, initiation of inspiratory flow requires inspiratory force to overcome PEEPi [9], which translates into increased inspiratory effort during the triggering phase. Ultimately, this increased effort may fail to trigger the ventilator, leading to ineffective triggering, one of the most frequent dyssynchronies [6]. In terms of gas exchange, patients with COPD have complex patterns of V/Q distributions: low V/Q regions that remain perfused, high V/Q regions, and mixed patterns. COPD patients often exhibit small amounts of shunt (typically less than 10% of cardiac output) [1].

Severe asthma exacerbation is characterized by a major increase in airway resistance due to bronchospasm, airway inflammation, and mucus. Expiratory flow is dramatically reduced with resultant major dynamic hyperinflation [10]. This leads to an increased risk of barotrauma and hemodynamic compromise. Hypoxemia in asthma is characterized by the presence of low V/Q units; hypoxemia is usually attenuated by compensatory redistribution of blood flow mediated by hypoxic vasoconstriction and changes in cardiac output [11].

10.2 Heart–Lung Interactions

The pathophysiological changes in the pulmonary system may have adverse effects on cardiac function. COPD is associated with pulmonary hypertension, increased pulmonary vascular resistance, right ventricle dilatation, and right ventricle hypertrophy. Both left ventricle systolic and left ventricle diastolic functions are often impaired in COPD patients [12]. These cardiac alterations are caused by dynamic hyperinflation and the large swings in negative intrathoracic pressure developed by the respiratory muscles to overcome the inspiratory elastic threshold caused by PEEPi and increased airway resistance. Dynamic hyperinflation is more detrimental to left ventricle hemodynamics than large swings in negative intrathoracic pressure [13]. Direct ventricular interaction and significant septal flattening appear to be responsible for reduced left ventricle end-diastolic volume and stroke volume [14]. Dynamic hyperinflation worsens the increase in right ventricular impedance (afterload effect), while large negative intrathoracic pressure swings increase the venous return to the right ventricle (preload effect). Both favor direct ventricular interaction with leftward shift of the septum.

Application of external PEEP up to values approaching PEEPi does not result in hemodynamic impairment in COPD [5]. Higher PEEP levels reduce cardiac index [15]. However, the effects of external PEEP on lung mechanics and hemodynamics depend on many factors, such as airway characteristics, lung volumes, intravascular volume status, vasomotor tone, etc., making the individual patient's response difficult to predict [16]. Finally, patients with COPD are at increased risk of difficult weaning and are susceptible to developing weaning-induced pulmonary edema in particular [17].

In patients with severe asthma, similar heart–lung interactions are observed. Because of the presence of an extremely severe hyperinflation, they may develop severe hypotension [18].

10.3   NIV in COPD

The utility of NIV in acute hypercapnic respiratory failure in COPD is well-established [19] and is included in the most recent international guidelines [20].

Selection criterion for initiation of NIV in patients with hypercapnic respiratory failure is a 2-step process that first determines whether the patient needs ventilatory assistance based on clinical and gas exchange criteria, and, if so, determine whether there are contraindications for NIV. NIV should be initiated as soon as the patient meets criteria for needing ventilatory assistance. Premature initiation wastes resources and increases intolerance rates, and delayed initiation permits patients to deteriorate to the point when intubation is unavoidable [21].

Indications for NIV are: tachypnea or increased work of breathing despite treatment with supplemental oxygen and nebulized bronchodilators; acute respiratory acidosis on blood gas analysis (pH < 7.35; PaCO2 > 45 mmHg); and mild alteration in mental status, which is attributed solely to hypercapnia [22]. Contraindications to NIV include hemodynamic instability or cardiopulmonary arrest; altered mental status not attributable to hypercapnia alone; poor secretion clearance, hemoptysis, active vomiting, upper gastrointestinal bleeding, or other airway compromise; recent facial surgery or trauma.

When compared with invasive mechanical ventilation, NIV has shown to have better outcomes and reduces risks of mortality and endotracheal intubation [23, 24]. Treatment with NIV is associated with a significant reduction in hospital length of stay on average, but this finding relates most often to patients with prolonged admissions [24].

NIV appears to improve acidosis within 1 h of initiation. There is no lower limit of pH below which a trial of NIV is inappropriate; however, the lower the pH, the greater the risk of failure, and patients must be very closely monitored with rapid access to endotracheal intubation and invasive ventilation if not improving [20]. Results of a systematic review appear generally consistent across both ICU and ward settings, and for patients admitted with more severe (pH < 7.30) or less severe (7.30–7.35) acidemia [24]. In a randomized study [25] comparing bilevel NIV to standard oxygen therapy in 52 patients with COPD with recent onset of shortness of breath and a pH > 7.30, NIV was poorly tolerated and there was no effect of NIV on intubation rate (8% in NIV arm and 7% in control arm) or mortality (4% in NIV arm and 7% in control arm), and there was a decrease in Borg dyspnea score at 1 h and on day 2 [25]. When one outlier was removed from the analysis, there was a statistically significant reduction in hospital length of stay with bilevel NIV compared with the control group (5 vs. 7 days) [25]. Three other studies [26–28], where the mean pH of included patients was only very mildly acidotic, did not show an advantage to bilevel NIV.

Given the lack of consistent evidence demonstrating benefit in those without acidosis and the potential for harm, the committee of the European Respiratory Society/American Thoracic Society practices guideline decided on a conditional recommendation against NIV in patients with hypercapnia who are not acidotic in the setting of a COPD exacerbation [20]. The main focus in hypercapnic patients with COPD who are not acidotic should be medical therapy and, most importantly, oxygen targeted to a saturation of 88–92% [29].

Need for endotracheal intubation was reduced by approximately two-thirds (64%) relative to usual care, equating to just five patients needing to be treated with NIV to potentially avoid intubation of one patient [24]. NIV reduces the sensation of dyspnea, the need for immediate intubation, ICU and probably hospital length of stay and improves survival [20], and both respiratory and non-respiratory infectious complications

[30, 31]. Use of NIV decreased the risk of mortality by 46% and decreased the risk of needing endotracheal intubation by 65% [24].

Two studies have compared bilevel NIV directly with invasive ventilation [32, 33]. In the study of Conti et al. [32], survival was similar in both groups, but in patients in whom NIV was successful the advantages included shorter duration of ICU and hospital stay, fewer complications, reduced need for de novo oxygen supplementation, and fewer hospital readmissions in the subsequent year. In the study of Jurjevic et al. [33], authors found that invasive ventilation was associated with more rapid improvement in physiological abnormalities in the first few hours, but was also associated with a longer total duration of ventilation and ICU stay. Mortality was similar in the two groups. Patients receiving NIV had fewer episodes of ventilator-associated pneumonia and less requirement for tracheostomy [33].

NIV may also be used as the only method for providing ventilatory support in patients who are not candidates for or decline invasive mechanical ventilation [20].

Non-invasive approaches use a variety of mechanisms to restore the balance of the supply and demand of breathing work [21]. CPAP alone reduces work of breathing in patients with severe COPD by counterbalancing auto-PEEP. Extrinsic PEEP (5–10 cm H2O) applied via a mask reduces the drop in pressure needed to create a negative pressure gradient and initiate air flow for the next breath. Pressure support also reduces the work of breathing by reducing the force inspiratory muscles must apply during inspiration [21]. The combination of PEEP and pressure support reduces diaphragmatic work in patients with COPD exacerbations more effectively than either one alone [34, 35], which helps to mitigate excessive work of breathing that leads to respiratory muscle fatigue and avoids worsening respiratory failure.

Another important step to consider is the timing of withdrawal of NIV. The 2016 BTS/ICS guideline states that NIV can be discontinued once the acidosis and hypercapnia have resolved, in a stepwise manner to avoid relapse of the hypercapnic failure [22], but there is scarce literature to support this approach compared with immediate withdrawal.

It is important to have markers to predict NIV failure prior to initiation of therapy, to either provide more intensive treatment in the form of invasive mechanical ventilation or allow a more conservative approach, if palliation is the most appropriate strategy. A higher APACHE II score (>20.5) at presentation, younger age, lower arterial bicarbonate levels, lower PaCO2, and high arterial lactate can predict failure of NIV [36, 37]. Others have identified baseline anemia [38], World Health Organization—Performance Status [38], and a nutritional risk screening 2002 score of greater than 3 [39]. Patients with evidence of diaphragmatic dysfunction at the time of admission are also more likely to suffer from NIV treatment failure [40]. Persistent tachycardia and acidosis 1 h after initiation of NIV also had an association with treatment failure [41].

The ERS/ATS guidelines recommend NIV for patients with ARF leading to acute or acute-on-chronic respiratory acidosis (pH $\leqslant$ 7.35) due to COPD exacerbation. Moreover, they recommend a trial of NIV in patients considered to require endotracheal intubation and mechanical ventilation, unless the patient is immediately deteriorating [20]. Rapid access to teams and resources capable of delivering invasive ventilation would therefore appear advisable for individuals considered appropriate for escalation of care when NIV is used.

10.4 NIV in Asthma

The main feature of acute asthma is a sudden and reversible episode of bronchoconstriction, leading to an increase in airways resistance that varies in severity. The acute change in mechanical load (mainly resistive) generates hyperinflation, increased respiratory muscle effort, and dyspnea. Hyperinflation also reduces respiratory muscle efficiency and thus the respiratory muscle pump may ultimately become exhausted, leading to hypercapnia [42].

NIV is used, together with conventional pharmacological treatment, with the aim to decrease the respiratory muscle work [43] that is much increased during the episodes of acute broncho-constriction, off-setting intrinsic PEEP [44, 45], alveolar recruitment, and to improve ventilation/perfusion mismatch [43, 46], decrease the sensation of dyspnea, and ultimately avoid intubation and invasive mechanical ventilation [20].

Studies have demonstrated a more rapid reversal of airway obstruction and a reduced need for hospitalization compared with standard therapy that could reflect a bronchodilator effect of positive airway pressure, but NIV has an unclear effect on mortality, intubation, or ICU length of stay [20].

Non-invasive ventilation provides a bronchodilatory effect with improvements in expiratory airflow. This has been observed as a direct effect of non-invasively applied CPAP after induced broncho-constriction [43, 47] or during acute exacerbations of asthma with applied bilevel positive airway pressure [48]. One small RCT found that NIV compared with sham treatment improved more the FEV1 after 3 h of therapy (FEV1%: 53.5 vs. 28.5; $P < 0.05$) [49]. In the study of Soma et al., patients with acute asthma of mild to moderate severity were randomly allocated to a NPPV ($n = 30$) or conventional oxygen therapy [48] ($n = 14$). Patients in the NPPV group were divided into two subgroups: a high- ($n = 16$) and a low-pressure group ($n = 14$) (inspiratory and expiratory pressures of 8 cm and 6 cm H2O and 6 cm and 4 cm H2O, respectively). The high-pressure NIV group had a 20% improvement in FEV1 over baseline compared with no improvement in controls treated with oxygen ($P < 0.05$). A third RCT enrolled subjects with severe airway obstruction and respiratory distress (average FEV1 of 21% predicted; frequency of 36 breaths/min) to receive NIV or conventional therapy with oxygen supplementation [50]. NIV use was associated with a trend toward more improvement in FEV1 in the first hour, less salbutamol use, and a shorter hospital length of stay [50]. Although not definitive, these data suggest that NIV could, thanks to a positive pressure-induced bronchodilator effect, help to improve air flow early on during severe asthma exacerbations.

During acute exacerbations of airway disease, the application of low-level externally applied PEEP helps reduce the pressure gradient between the distal and central airways and possibly the level of intrinsic PEEP itself that is established during dynamic hyperinflation [43]. As a consequence, the reduction in intrathoracic pressure necessary for initiation of inspiratory airflow is less, which helps to off-load the inspiratory muscle work and improve their efficiency [43]. This effect is likely maximal as extrinsic PEEP is increased to levels close to, but ideally not exceeding, intrinsic PEEP [51]. Moreover, the addition of a pressure support, or inspiratory positive airway pressure (IPAP) in the NIV setting, helps to further unload the inspiratory muscles while augmenting ventilation [52].

Ventilation/perfusion inequality, likely due to obstructed peripheral airways, is also a significant contributing factor to respiratory compromise in acute asthma [43]. The utilization of external PEEP or EPAP has demonstrated improvements in ventilation/perfusion matching and gas exchange and represents another potential benefit of NIV [43].

Great caution is advised, however, when using high levels of PEEP in asthma. It has been suggested that externally applied PEEP should not be used indiscriminately in patients with obstructive airways disease, but rather in a specific subset in whom expiratory flow limitation, dynamic airway compression, and dyspnea are the primary problems [53]. In this setting, external PEEP or the non-invasive equivalent of EPAP/CPAP may possibly be used safely without significant increases in lung volume so long as set values do not exceed the previously established level of intrinsic PEEP [51]. This scenario, however, is more readily applicable in patients with COPD and perhaps less so in asthmatic patients, where there is bronchospasm but without the same degree of dynamic airway compression [43]. In the setting of asthma where expiratory airflow is limited by a fixed resistance, rather than dynamic airway collapse, application of external PEEP may potentially immediately translate into hyperinflation at any given level of PEEP/EPAP and therefore cause harm to the patient [43].

A Cochrane review considered NIV for asthma promising but controversial [54] and the European Respiratory Society/American Thoracic Society guideline made no recommendation due to a lack of evidence [20].

NIV can be considered to treat acute severe asthma and may be useful to avoid intubation in status asthmaticus, although more studies are clearly needed to test this possibility and to assess the clinical utility of its apparent early bronchodilator effect. In the meantime, caution should be exercised because some patients with severe asthma can deteriorate rapidly and develop very-severe obstruction, which makes ventilation difficult, even via the invasive route [21]. However, if a patient's condition is severe enough that endotracheal intubation is inevitable, this should be performed immediately and without delay. It is therefore important that a trial of NIV is performed in an ICU setting by experienced personnel where endotracheal intubation can be performed quickly.

References

1. Demoule A, et al. How to ventilate obstructive and asthmatic patients. Intensive Care Med. 2020;46(12):2436–49. https://doi.org/10.1007/s00134-020-06291-0.
2. Peñuelas O, et al. Inter-country variability over time in the mortality of mechanically ventilated patients. Intensive Care Med. 2020;46(3):444–53. https://doi.org/10.1007/s00134-019-05867-9.
3. Pendergraft TB, et al. Rates and characteristics of intensive care unit admissions and intubations among asthma-related hospitalizations. Ann Allergy Asthma Immunol. 2004;93(1):29–35. https://doi.org/10.1016/S1081-1206(10)61444-5.
4. Vassilakopoulos T, Toumpanakis D, Mancebo J. What's new about pulmonary hyperinflation in mechanically ventilated critical patients. Intensive Care Med. 2020;46(12):2381–4. https://doi.org/10.1007/s00134-020-06105-3.
5. Junhasavasdikul D, et al. Expiratory flow limitation during mechanical ventilation. Chest. 2018;154(4):948–62. https://doi.org/10.1016/j.chest.2018.01.046.
6. Vassilakopoulos T. Understanding wasted/ineffective efforts in mechanically ventilated COPD patients using the campbell diagram. Intensive Care Med. 2008;34(7):1336–9. https://doi.org/10.1007/s00134-008-1095-7.
7. Marini JJ, Jaber S. Dynamic predictors of VILI risk: beyond the driving pressure. Intensive Care Med. 2016;42(10):1597–600. https://doi.org/10.1007/s00134-016-4534-x.
8. Marini JJ. Dynamic hyperinflation and auto-positive end-expiratory pressure lessons learned over 30 years. Am J Respir Crit Care Med. 2011;184(7):756–62. https://doi.org/10.1164/rccm.201102-0226PP.
9. Smith TC, Marini JJ. Impact of PEEP on lung mechanics and work of breathing in severe airflow obstruction. J Appl Physiol. 1988;65(4):1488–99. https://doi.org/10.1152/jappl.1988.65.4.1488.
10. Oddo M, Feihl F, Schaller MD, Perret C. Management of mechanical ventilation in acute severe asthma: practical aspects. Intensive Care Med. 2006;32(4):501–10. https://doi.org/10.1007/s00134-005-0045-x.
11. Young IH, Bye PTP. Gas exchange in disease: asthma, chronic obstructive pulmonary disease, cystic fibrosis, and interstitial lung disease. Compr Physiol. 2011;1(2):663–97. https://doi.org/10.1002/cphy.c090012.
12. Abroug F, et al. Association of left-heart dysfunction with severe exacerbation of chronic obstructive pulmonary disease: diagnostic performance of cardiac biomarkers. Am J Respir Crit Care Med. 2006;174(9):990–6. https://doi.org/10.1164/rccm.200603-380OC.
13. Cheyne WS, Williams AM, Harper MI, Eves ND. Heart-lung interaction in a model of COPD: importance of lung volume and direct ventricular interaction. Am J Physiol Heart Circ Physiol. 2016;311(6):H1367–74. https://doi.org/10.1152/ajpheart.00458.2016.
14. Cheyne WS, Gelinas JC, Eves ND. Hemodynamic effects of incremental lung hyperinflation. Am J Physiol Heart Circ Physiol. 2018;315(3):H474–81. https://doi.org/10.1152/ajpheart.00229.2018.
15. Dambrosio M, et al. Effects of positive end-expiratory pressure on right ventricular function in COPD patients during acute ventilatory failure. Intensive Care Med. 1996;22(9):923–32. https://doi.org/10.1007/BF02044117.
16. Georgopulos D, Giannouli E, Patakas D. Effects of extrinsic positive end-expiratory pressure on mechanically ventilated patients with chronic obstructive pulmonary disease and dynamic hyperinflation. Intensive Care Med. 1993;19(4):197–203. https://doi.org/10.1007/BF01694770.
17. Liu J, et al. Cardiac dysfunction induced by weaning from mechanical ventilation: incidence, risk factors, and effects of fluid removal. Crit Care. 2016;20(1):369. https://doi.org/10.1186/s13054-016-1533-9.
18. Corbridge TC, Hall JB. The assessment and management of adults with status asthmaticus. Am J Respir Crit Care Med. 1995;151(5):1296–316. https://doi.org/10.1164/ajrccm.151.5.7735578.
19. Chandra D, et al. Outcomes of noninvasive ventilation for acute exacerbations of chronic obstructive pulmonary disease in the United States, 1998-2008. Am J

Respir Crit Care Med. 2012;185(2):152–9. https://doi.org/10.1164/rccm.201106-1094OC.

20. Rochwerg B, et al. Official ERS/ATS clinical practice guidelines: noninvasive ventilation for acute respiratory failure. Eur Respir J. 2017;50(2):1602426. https://doi.org/10.1183/13993003.02426-2016.

21. Hill NS, Spoletini G, Schumaker G, Garpestad E. Noninvasive ventilatory support for acute hypercapnic respiratory failure. Respir Care. 2019;64(6):647–57. https://doi.org/10.4187/respcare.06931.

22. Davidson AC, et al. BTS/ICS guideline for the ventilatory management of acute hypercapnic respiratory failure in adults. Thorax. 2016;71 Suppl 2:ii1–35. https://doi.org/10.1136/thoraxjnl-2015-208209.

23. Lindenauer PK, et al. Outcomes associated with invasive and noninvasive ventilation among patients hospitalized with exacerbations of chronic obstructive pulmonary disease. JAMA Intern Med. 2014;174(12):1982–93. https://doi.org/10.1001/jamainternmed.2014.5430.

24. Osadnik CR, et al. Non-invasive ventilation for the management of acute hypercapnic respiratory failure due to exacerbation of chronic obstructive pulmonary disease. Cochrane Database Syst Rev. 2017;7(7):CD004104. https://doi.org/10.1002/14651858.CD004104.pub4.

25. Keenan SP, Powers CE, McCormack DG. Noninvasive positive-pressure ventilation in patients with milder chronic obstructive pulmonary disease exacerbations: a randomized controlled trial. Respir Care. 2005;50(5):610–6.

26. Barbé F, et al. Noninvasive ventilatory support does not facilitate recovery from acute respiratory failure in chronic obstructive pulmonary disease. Eur Respir J. 1996;9(6):1240–5. https://doi.org/10.1183/09031936.96.09061240.

27. Bardi G, et al. Nasal ventilation in COPD exacerbations: early and late results of a prospective, controlled study. Eur Respir J. 2000;15(1):98–104. https://doi.org/10.1034/j.1399-3003.2000.15a18.x.

28. Wood KA, Lewis L, Von Harz B, Kollef MH. The use of noninvasive positive pressure ventilation in the emergency department: results of a randomized clinical trial. Chest. 1998;113(5):1339–46. https://doi.org/10.1378/chest.113.5.1339.

29. O'Driscoll BR, Howard LS, Davison AG. BTS guideline for emergency oxygen use in adult patients. Thorax. 2008;63 Suppl 6:vi1–68. https://doi.org/10.1136/thx.2008.102947.

30. Girou E, Brun-Buisson C, Taillé S, Lemaire F, Brochard L. Secular trends in nosocomial infections and mortality associated with noninvasive ventilation in patients with exacerbation of COPD and pulmonary edema. J Am Med Assoc. 2003;290(22):2985–91. https://doi.org/10.1001/jama.290.22.2985.

31. Girou E, et al. Association of noninvasive ventilation with nosocomial infections and survival in critically ill patients. J Am Med Assoc. 2000;284(18):2361–7. https://doi.org/10.1001/jama.284.18.2361.

32. Conti G, et al. Noninvasive vs. conventional mechanical ventilation in patients with chronic obstructive pulmonary disease after failure of medical treatment in the ward: a randomized trial. Intensive Care Med. 2002;28(12):1701–7. https://doi.org/10.1007/s00134-002-1478-0.

33. Jurjević M, et al. Mechanical ventilation in chronic obstructive pulmonary disease patients, noninvasive vs. invasive method (randomized prospective study). Coll Antropol. 2009;33(3):791–7.

34. Kramer N, Meyer TJ, Meharg J, Cece RD, Hill NS. Randomized, prospective trial of noninvasive positive pressure ventilation in acute respiratory failure. Am J Respir Crit Care Med. 1995;151(6):1799–806. https://doi.org/10.1164/ajrccm.151.6.7767523.

35. Appendini L, et al. Physiologic effects of positive end-expiratory pressure and mask pressure support during exacerbations of chronic obstructive pulmonary disease. Am J Respir Crit Care Med. 1994;149(5):1069–76. https://doi.org/10.1164/ajrccm.149.5.8173743.

36. Corrêa TD, et al. Performance of noninvasive ventilation in acute respiratory failure in critically ill patients: a prospective, observational, cohort study. BMC Pulm Med. 2015;15:144. https://doi.org/10.1186/s12890-015-0139-3.

37. Conti V, et al. Predictors of outcome for patients with severe respiratory failure requiring non invasive mechanical ventilation. Eur Rev Med Pharmacol Sci. 2015;19(20):3855–60.

38. Mydin HH, Murphy S, Clague H, Sridharan K, Taylor IK. Anemia and performance status as prognostic markers in acute hypercapnic respiratory failure due to chronic obstructive pulmonary disease. Int J COPD. 2013;8:151–7. https://doi.org/10.2147/COPD.S39403.

39. Cui J, et al. Nutritional risk screening 2002 as a predictor of outcome during general ward-based noninvasive ventilation in chronic obstructive pulmonary disease with respiratory failure. Med Sci Monit. 2015;21:2786–93. https://doi.org/10.12659/MSM.894191.

40. Antenora F, et al. Prevalence and outcomes of diaphragmatic dysfunction assessed by ultrasound technology during acute exacerbation of COPD: a pilot study. Respirology. 2017;22(2):338–44. https://doi.org/10.1111/resp.12916.

41. Ko BS, et al. Early failure of noninvasive ventilation in chronic obstructive pulmonary disease with acute hypercapnic respiratory failure. Intern Emerg Med. 2015;10(7):855–60. https://doi.org/10.1007/s11739-015-1293-6.

42. Leatherman J. Mechanical ventilation for severe asthma. Chest. 2015;147(6):1671–80. https://doi.org/10.1378/chest.14-1733.

43. Pallin M, Naughton MT. Noninvasive ventilation in acute asthma. J Crit Care. 2014;11(5):727–32. https://doi.org/10.1016/j.jcrc.2014.03.011.

44. Sassoon CSH, Light RW, Lodia R, Sieck GC, Mahutte CK. Pressure-time product during continuous positive airway pressure, pressure support ventilation, and

T-piece during weaning from mechanical ventilation. Am Rev Respir Dis. 1991;143(3):469–75. https://doi.org/10.1164/ajrccm/143.3.469.

45. Sydow M, et al. Effect of low-level PEEP on inspiratory work of breathing in intubated patients, both with healthy lungs and with COPD. Intensive Care Med. 1995;21(11):887–95. https://doi.org/10.1007/BF01712329.

46. Meduri GU, Cook TR, Turner RE, Cohen M, Leeper KV. Noninvasive positive pressure ventilation in status asthmaticus. Chest. 1996;110(3):767–74. https://doi.org/10.1378/chest.110.3.767.

47. Wang CH, et al. Differential effects of nasal continuous positive airway pressure on reversible or fixed upper and lower airway obstruction. Eur Respir J. 1996;9(5):952–9. https://doi.org/10.1183/09031936.96.09050952.

48. Soma T, Hino M, Kida K, Kudoh S. A prospective and randomized study for improvement of acute asthma by non-invasive positive pressure ventilation (NPPV). Intern Med. 2008;47(6):493–501. https://doi.org/10.2169/internalmedicine.47.0429.

49. Soroksky A, Stav D, Shpirer I. A pilot prospective, randomized, placebo-controlled trial of bilevel positive airway pressure in acute asthmatic attack. Chest. 2003;123(4):1018–25. https://doi.org/10.1378/chest.123.4.1018.

50. Gupta D, Nath A, Agarwal R, Behera D. A prospective randomized controlled trial on the efficacy of noninvasive ventilation in severe acute asthma. Respir Care. 2010;55(5):536–43.

51. Guerin C, Milic-Emili J, Fournier G. Effect of PEEP on work of breathing in mechanically ventilated COPD patients. Intensive Care Med. 2000;26(9):1207–14. https://doi.org/10.1007/s001340051339.

52. Tokioka H, et al. Effectiveness of pressure support ventilation for mechanical ventilatory support in patients with status asthmaticus. Acta Anaesthesiol Scand. 1992;36(1):5–9. https://doi.org/10.1111/j.1399-6576.1992.tb03413.x.

53. Marini JJ. Should PEEP be used in airflow obstruction? Am Rev Respir Dis. 1989;140(1):1–3. https://doi.org/10.1164/ajrccm/140.1.1.

54. Lim WJ, et al. Non-invasive positive pressure ventilation for treatment of respiratory failure due to severe acute exacerbations of asthma. Cochrane Database Syst Rev. 2012;12:CD004360. https://doi.org/10.1002/14651858.cd004360.pub4.

S. Nappi and A. Marra

Content

The devices used for NIV are applied externally, are minimally invasive, and give pressure and flow to upper airways; they include high flow nasal oxygen, helmet, full face mask, and oronasal mask. NIV is well-known therapy for acute respiratory failure, especially in patients with hypercapnia and cardiogenic pulmonary edema. On contrary, NIV treatment is still debated in case of acute hypoxemic respiratory failure (AHRF) and its subset, acute respiratory distress syndrome (ARDS) [1].

We can define an ARDS when we found a bilateral pulmonary infiltrates on chest X-ray, and hypoxemia, non-completely explained by fluid overload and/or cardiac dysfunction, assessed with a positive end-respiratory pressure (PEEP) of at least 5 cm^2 H2O [2].

Hypoxemia is classified by the PaO2/FiO2 ratio: it is mild in case of a ratio equal to 201–300 mmHg, moderate if equal to 101–200 mmHg, and severe if minor to 100 mmHg [3]. Studies demonstrated that in case of mild hypoxemia,

non-invasive oxygenation supports can prevent endotracheal intubation compared with standard oxygen therapy [4], while in case of moderate to severe hypoxemia, its efficacy is still unclear, but if intubation is required after NIV support, the mortality risk is increased [5].

The use of NIV reduces the risk of the complications related to sedation, endotracheal intubation, and invasive ventilation [4], the risk of delirium [1], and prevent diaphragm dysfunction and atrophy [6, 7]; it keeps constant the cardiac preloading and cardiac output [8, 9] and increases ventilation/perfusion mismatch [10–12]. From a physiological point of view, in a patient treated with non-invasive ventilation, breathing and oxygenation may improve thanks to the alveolar recruitment, ameliorating the dyspnea, and consequently improving clinical outcomes avoiding the need for invasive ventilation.

However, the patient's inspiratory effort, the high tidal volume, the tachypnea, combined with the NIV treatment, can lead to high transpulmonary pressure swings, lung overstretch and thus, patient self-inflicted lung injury (PSILI) [13–16]. According to physiology of ARDS, the presence of edema, alveolar flooding, and atelectasis causes an inhomogeneous inspiratory force

S. Nappi · A. Marra (✉)
Unit of Anesthesia and Intensive Care, Department of Neurosciences, Reproductive and Odontostomatological Sciences, University of Naples "Federico II", Naples, Italy

© The Author(s), under exclusive license to Springer Nature Switzerland AG 2023
G. Servillo, M. Vargas (eds.), *Non-invasive Mechanical Ventilation in Critical Care, Anesthesiology and Palliative Care*, https://doi.org/10.1007/978-3-031-36510-2_11

across lungs tissues, increasing the worsening of inflammation and the overstretching [13]. This mechanism shifts the lung gases from anterior zone to posterior region, causing the so-called *pendelluft* phenomenon [17, 18]. The huge inspiratory effort causes a pleural pressure negative deflection, increasing transmural capillary pressure and exacerbating interstitial and alveolar edema [19]. This inhomogeneous pressure in various lung regions may cause an injury of the diaphragm, affecting short- and long-term clinical outcomes [20, 21]. These are the main reasons why patients are intubated after NIV support; they have an increased mortality risk [22, 23]. Moreover, it is clear that the delayed intubation also affects the clinical outcome, whereas it improves when non-invasive ventilation allows to avoid invasive ventilation [1].

Many studies were conducted to find evidence in support of or against NIV in ARDS. Frat et al. [24] found that in moderate to severe acute hypoxemic respiratory failure, treatment with high-flow nasal oxygen (HFNO) or other NIV interfaces did not result in significant different intubation rates, even if patients treated with high-flow nasal oxygen (HFNO) had a slightly lower risk of intubation compared to patients treated with facemask NIV. It is important to note that sedative and opioid analgesia often increases the NIV failure rate.

Patel et al. [25] showed that there was a reduction in intubation rate and mortality in patients treated with helmet compared to those treated with facemask (18.2% vs. 61.5%), bringing the attention to the importance of NIV interface. The single center trial was interrupted early for efficacy and the lower intubation rate was associated with more ventilator-free day and lower mortality. This study emphasizes the importance of protective ventilation during NIV therapy. This includes low tidal volume, low plateau pressures, and high PEEP values. Indeed, the necessity of a huge tidal volume may be a marker of NIV failure (threshold tidal 9.5 mL/kg) and it suggests requirement for invasive ventilation.

Ferreyro et al. [4] compared both HFNO and helmet NIV and facemask NIV showing in all cases a reduction in the risk of endotracheal intubation. Bellani et al. [26] (lung-safe study) underlined that the NIV failure was strongly correlated with the severity of ARDS and the magnitude of the decrease in the PaO2/FiO2 ratio was an independent predictor of mortality.

In conclusion, NIV seems effective in mild-to-moderate hypoxemia (PaO2/FiO2 > 150 mmHg), while no conclusive evidence has been found in the management through NIV of moderate to severe (PaO2/FiO2 < 150 mmHg) hypoxemia [1]. Certainly, some strategies are available to limit the PSILI and to increase the NIV efficacy [27]. Propofol and benzodiazepines have shown to reduce respiratory effort, so their use during NIV treatment is suggested [28], while it is known that opioid reduces respiratory rate, increasing the risk of apnea and dyspnea and so during NIV therapy must be avoided [29, 30]. The application of high level of PEEP (10–15 cm H2O) improves the ventilation homogeneity and prevent *pendelluft* phenomenon, also protecting the diaphragm from injuries [31, 32].

Each technique providing non-invasive ventilation has its benefits and its pitfalls [1]. HFNO enhances comfort, provides positive airway pressure (up to 4 cm H2O), makes a washout of nasopharyngeal dead space, and reduces inspiratory effort. However, the main disadvantage is the small amount of PEEP delivered.

The benefits of facemask are providing PEEP to allow alveolar recruitment and PS (only for PSV) to unload inspiratory muscles. It allows to monitor tidal volume (only PSV) too. The pitfalls are skin ulcer and air leaks, accompanied therefore by the difficulty in delivery of high PEEP. Moreover, the full inspiratory synchronization rhythm may increase PL swings and the poor tolerability causes many treatment interruptions.

Among NIV interfaces, helmet provides the highest level of PEEP to allow alveolar recruitment and to enhance ventilator homogeneity. It is a continuous treatment with good tolerability; it provides PS (only for PSV) to reduce inspiratory effort and to prevent positive PL swings. However, the impossibility to measure tidal volume and the occurrence of upper limbs edema, with possible vasal thrombosis, are concerning disadvantages [1].

The monitoring of patient under NIV therapy must be very frequent in order to assess in time the early signs of NIV failure and to avoid delayed intubation [33–35]. Pulse oximetry, PaO2/FiO2, inspiratory efforts, and respiratory rate should be monitored continuously when possible; pay attention to the occurrence of moderate-severe hypoxia and the abrupt necessity to endotracheal intubation. Some index can help physicians to predict the outcome of NIV therapy and the risk of endotracheal intubation.

The ROX index [36] defined as the ratio between SpO2/FiO2 and respiratory rate accurately predicted the outcome of HFNO. Repeated assessment of the HACOR scale (which includes heart rate, acidosis, consciousness, oxygenation, and respiratory rate) allows dynamic monitoring of the risk of endotracheal intubation during face-mask NIV [37]. To date, no validated score exists to predict failure during helmet NIV. We can conclude this chapter, with this home-message: NIV is not recommended as first-line therapy in ARDS management, but may benefit those who do not require immediate intubation with mild to moderate hypoxemia [1].

References

1. Grieco LD, et al. Non-invasive ventilatory support and high-flow nasal oxygen as first-line treatment of acute hypoxemic respiratory failure and ARDS. Intensive Care Med. 2021;47:851–66. https://doi.org/10.1007/s00134-021-06459-2.
2. Definition Task Force ARDS, Ranieri VM, Rubenfeld GD, et al. Acute respiratory distress syndrome: the Berlin Definition. JAMA. 2012;307:2526–33. https://doi.org/10.1001/jama.2012.5669.
3. Pham T, Pesenti A, Bellani G, et al. Outcome of acute Hypoxaemic respiratory failure. Eur Respir J, Insights from the Lung Safe Study. 2020;57(6):2003317. https://doi.org/10.1183/13993003.03317-2020.
4. Ferreyro BL, Angriman F, Munshi L, et al. Association of noninvasive oxygenation strategies with all-cause mortality in adults with acute hypoxemic respiratory failure. JAMA. 2020;324:57. https://doi.org/10.1001/jama.2020.9524.
5. Rochwerg B, Einav S, Chaudhuri D, et al. The role for high flow nasal cannula as a respiratory support strategy in adults: a clinical practice guideline. Intensive Care Med. 2020;46:2226–37. https://doi.org/10.1007/s00134-020-06312-y.
6. Squadrone V, Coha M, Cerutti E, et al. Continuous positive airway pressure for treatment of postoperative hypoxemia: a randomized controlled trial. JAMA. 2005;293:589–95. https://doi.org/10.1001/jama.293.5.589.
7. Sassoon CSH, Zhu E, Caiozzo VJ. Assist-control mechanical ventilation attenuates ventilator-induced diaphragmatic dysfunction. Am J Respir Crit Care Med. 2004;170:626–32. https://doi.org/10.1164/rccm.200401-042OC.
8. Qvist J, Pontoppidan H, Wilson RS, et al. Hemodynamic responses to mechanical ventilation with PEEP: the effect of hypervolemia. Anesthesiology. 1975;42:45–55. https://doi.org/10.1097/00000542-197501000-00009.
9. Repesse X, Charron C, Vieillard-Baron A. Right ventricular failure in acute lung injury and acute respiratory distress syndrome. Minerva Anestesiol. 2012;78:941–8.
10. Wrigge H, Zinserling J, Neumann P, et al. Spontaneous breathing improves lung aeration in oleic acid-induced lung injury. Anesthesiology. 2003;99:376–84. https://doi.org/10.1097/00000542-200308000-00019.
11. Ferrari S, Orlandi M, Avella M, et al. Effects of hydration on plasma concentrations of methotrexate in patients with osteosarcoma treated with high doses of methotrexate. Minerva Med. 1992;83:289–93. https://doi.org/10.1097/01.ccm.0000163226.34868.0a.
12. Putensen C, Zech S, Wrigge H, et al. Long-term effects of spontaneous breathing during ventilatory support in patients with acute lung injury. Am J Respir Crit Care Med. 2001;164:43–9. https://doi.org/10.1164/ajrccm.164.1.2001078.
13. Carteaux G, Millan-Guilarte T, De Prost N, et al. Failure of noninvasive ventilation for de novo acute hypoxemic respiratory failure: role of tidal volume. Crit Care Med. 2016;44:282–90. https://doi.org/10.1097/CCM.0000000000001379.
14. Frat J-P, Ragot S, Coudroy R, et al. Predictors of intubation in patients with acute hypoxemic respiratory failure treated with a noninvasive oxygenation strategy. Crit Care Med. 2018;46:208–15. https://doi.org/10.1097/CCM.0000000000002818.
15. Yoshida T, Fujino Y, Amato MBP, Kavanagh BP. Fifty years of research in ARDS. Spontaneous breathing during mechanical ventilation. Risks, mechanisms, and management. Am J Respir Crit Care Med. 2017;195:985–92. https://doi.org/10.1164/rccm.201604-0748CP.
16. Brochard L, Slutsky A, Pesenti A. Mechanical ventilation to minimize progression of lung injury in acute respiratory failure. Am J Respir Crit Care Med. 2017;195:438–42. https://doi.org/10.1164/rccm.201605-1081CP.
17. Yoshida T, Torsani V, Gomes S, et al. Spontaneous effort causesoccult pendelluft during mechanical ventilation. Am J Respir Crit CareMed. 2013;188:1420–7. https://doi.org/10.1164/rccm.201303-0539OC.

18. Yoshida T, Roldan R, Beraldo MA, et al. Spontaneous effort during mechanical ventilation: maximal injury with less positive end-expiratory pressure. Crit Care Med. 2016;44:e678–88. https://doi.org/10.1097/CCM.0000000000001649.

19. Bhattacharya M, Kallet RH, Ware LB, Matthay MA. Negative-pressure pulmonary edema. Chest. 2016;150:927–33. https://doi.org/10.1016/j.chest.2016.03.043.

20. Goligher EC, Jonkman AH, Dianti J, et al. Clinical strategies for implementing lung and diaphragm-protective ventilation: avoiding insufficient and excessive effort. Intensive Care Med. 2020;46:2314–26. https://doi.org/10.1007/s00134-020-06288-9.

21. Goligher EC, Brochard LJ, Reid WD, et al. Diaphragmatic myotrauma: a mediator of prolonged ventilation and poor patient outcomes in acute respiratory failure. Lancet Respir Med. 2019;7:90–8. https://doi.org/10.1016/S2213-2600(18)30366-7.

22. Carrillo A, Gonzalez-Diaz G, Ferrer M, et al. Non-invasive ventilation in community-acquired pneumonia and severe acute respiratory failure. Intensive Care Med. 2012;38:458–66. https://doi.org/10.1007/s00134-012-2475-6.

23. Demoule A, Girou E, Richard J-C, et al. Benefits and risks of success or failure of noninvasive ventilation. Intensive Care Med. 2006;32:1756–65. https://doi.org/10.1007/s00134-006-0324-1.

24. Frat J-P, Thille AW, Mercat A, et al. High-flow oxygen through nasal cannula in acute hypoxemic respiratory failure. N Engl J Med. 2015;372:2185–96. https://doi.org/10.1056/NEJMoa1503326.

25. Nava S, Hill N. Non-invasive ventilation in acute respiratory failure. Lancet. 2009;374:250–9. https://doi.org/10.1016/S0140-6736(09)60496-7.

26. Bellani G, Laffey JG, Pham T, et al. Noninvasive ventilation of patients with acute respiratory distress syndrome. Insights from the LUNG SAFE study. Am J Respir Crit Care Med. 2017;195:67–77. https://doi.org/10.1164/rccm.201606-1306OC.

27. Goligher EC, Dres M, Patel BK, et al. Lung- and diaphragm-protective ventilation. Am J Respir Crit Care Med. 2020;202:950–61. https://doi.org/10.1164/rccm.202003-0655CP.

28. Vaschetto R, Cammarota G, Colombo D, et al. Effects of propofol on patient-ventilator synchrony and interaction during pressure support ventilation and neurally adjusted ventilatory assist. Crit Care Med. 2014;42:74–82. https://doi.org/10.1097/CCM.0b013e31829e53dc.

29. Pattinson KTS. Opioids and the control of respiration. Br J Anaesth. 2008;100:747–58. https://doi.org/10.1093/bja/aen094.

30. Chanques G, Constantin J-M, Devlin JW, et al. Analgesia and sedation in patients with ARDS. Intensive Care Med. 2020;46:2342–56. https://doi.org/10.1007/s00134-020-06307-9.

31. Morais CCA, Koyama Y, Yoshida T, et al. High positive end expiratory pressure renders spontaneous effort noninjurious. Am J Respir Crit Care Med. 2018;197:1285–96. https://doi.org/10.1164/rccm.201706-1244OC.

32. Evans CL, Hill AV. The relation of length to tension development and heat production on contraction in muscle. J Physiol. 1914;49:10–6. https://doi.org/10.1113/jphysiol.1914.sp001684.

33. Tobin MJ, Laghi F, Jubran A. Why COVID-19 silent hypoxemia is baffling to physicians. Am J Respir Crit Care Med. 2020;202:356–60. https://doi.org/10.1164/rccm.202006-2157CP.

34. Antonelli M, Conti G, Esquinas A, et al. A multiple-center survey on the use in clinical practice of noninvasive ventilation as a first-line intervention for acute respiratory distress syndrome. Crit Care Med. 2007;35:18–25. https://doi.org/10.1097/01.CCM.0000251821.44259.F3.

35. Antonelli M, Conti G, Moro ML, et al. Predictors of failure of noninvasive positive pressure ventilation in patients with acute hypoxemic respiratory failure: a multi-center study. Intensive Care Med. 2001;27:1718–28. https://doi.org/10.1007/s00134-001-1114-4.

36. Roca O, Caralt B, Messika J, et al. An index combining respiratory rate and oxygenation to predict outcome of nasal high-flow therapy. Am J Respir Crit Care Med. 2019;199:1368–76. https://doi.org/10.1164/rccm.201803-0589OC.

37. Duan J, Han X, Bai L, et al. Assessment of heart rate, acidosis, consciousness, oxygenation, and respiratory rate to predict noninvasive ventilation failure in hypoxemic patients. Intensive Care Med. 2017;43:192–9. https://doi.org/10.1007/s00134-016-4601-3.

Giuseppe Servillo, Pasquale Buonanno,
Serena Nappi, Francesco Squillacioti,
and Ivana Capuano

Contents

12.1 Introduction

Nowadays, after 3 years from the beginning of the actual pandemic, the best ventilatory management of acute respiratory failure in COVID-19 disease is still unknown. Initially, in the WHO guidelines of 2020, it has been reported that there are no indications in the use of non-invasive ventilation (NIV) in case of hypoxemic respiratory failure other than cardiogenic pulmonary edema and postoperative respiratory failure and in case of viral diseases. It has been also suggested that patients receiving NIV should be hemodynamically stable, conscious and strictly controlled, monitored, and cured by expert staff in emergency tracheal intubation [1].

Indeed, the early reports of Chinese physicians who managed the first cases of COVID patients pointed out the importance of an early intubation in order not to delay invasive ventilation [2].

In the pre-COVID era, NIV was commonly used in short-term life-threatening respiratory diseases such as type 2 respiratory failure, while there is no sufficient data to support the use of NIV in type 1 respiratory failure; however, during the pandemic, continuous positive airway pressure (CPAP) gained an important role in facing the early phases of COVID-19, preventing further lung injuries, risk of invasive ventilation, and improving oxygenation [2]. In order to administer a CPAP, a tight-fitting mask or a hood (sealed system) is necessary that delivers a mixture of oxygen and air by a positive pressure, thus

G. Servillo · P. Buonanno (✉) · S. Nappi ·
F. Squillacioti · I. Capuano
Department of Neurosciences and Reproductive and
Odontostomatological Sciences, University of Naples
"Federico II", Naples, Italy

© The Author(s), under exclusive license to Springer Nature Switzerland AG 2023
G. Servillo, M. Vargas (eds.), *Non-invasive Mechanical Ventilation in Critical Care, Anesthesiology
and Palliative Care*, https://doi.org/10.1007/978-3-031-36510-2_12

supporting patient breaths. Specifically, some studies claimed that the right setting for COVID-19 disease is a pressure of 10 cm H2O and a fraction of inspired oxygen of 60%, while target SpO2 should be 92–96% in patients without chronic lung diseases, 88–92% in ones with chronic lung diseases. NIV and high flow nasal oxygen (HFNO) also have a bridging role after extubation [2].

Notably, CPAP used in COVID disease is cCPAP, while iCPAP has not a major clinical effect on ARDS. The cCPAP must be settled with a pressure of 10–12 cm H2O or higher and the positive effect should be noticeable immediately after its application with a decrease in respiratory rate and an improvement in gas exchange [3].

Bilevel positive airway pressure (BiPAP) is used in COVID patients who have comorbidities such as COPD, taking care of the increased risk of barotrauma and pneumothorax. BIPAP requires the setting of an inspiratory positive airway pressure (IPAP), an expiratory positive airway pressure (EPAP), and a pressure support can be delivered. The latter should be at least equal to 8 cm H2O in COVID disease and it is to be set in order to achieve an adequate tidal volume. However, BIPAP is still considered an experimental ventilation in COVID 19 [2, 3].

CPAP and BiPAP need time and continuous application to be effective, even if sometimes the tight-fitting mask and the hood can be a challenge for the patient compliance. The noise produced by the air flow, claustrophobia, abrasions, sores and edema of the cornea, and conjunctiva are some of the disadvantages of the mask while the hood can also cause discomfort in the armpit; in addition, vomiting and the necessity in some patients to frequently aspirate oral and nasal secretions can make NIV administration more difficult. The assessment of pulse, vital and neurological signs, saturation, and a first ABG within 1 h from the beginning of the treatment and repeated within four and 12 h are always recommended. Moreover, NIV produces high intrathoracic pressure, and in patients hemodynamically unstable, can cause a reduced venous return, thus compromising cardiovascular conditions [2].

12.2 NIV Indications and Modifications in Covid-19: Benefits and Advantages

Lung recruitment, during hypoxemia in COVID 19, in order to prevent alveoli to collapse, may be achieved either with prone positioning or varying positions and/or positive airway pressure (e.g., CPAP or BiPAP). The prone position helps the recruitment of non-dependent lung tissue while CPAP directly promotes alveolar inflation. Non-invasive Ventilation (NIV) refers to the application of mechanical ventilatory support using a nasal, oronasal, full-face device, or a helmet. Only selected patients are candidable for NIV and HFNO, such as those with a ceiling of treatment or patients presenting with hypercapnic respiratory failure. It is also indicated for patients who do not respond to conventional oxygen therapy [3]. In particular, treatment with helmet non-invasive ventilation showed to improve oxygenation and reduce inspiratory effort as compared with HFNO. These benefits have led to reduced intubation rate among patients compared with patients receiving NIV by face mask. The helmet was also associated with increased ventilator-free days and significantly reduced intensive care unit (ICU) length of stay and 90-day mortality [4].

As highlighted in the HENIVOT RCT, the rate of endotracheal intubation was significantly lower in the subjects who were treated with helmet non-invasive ventilation than with the HFNO (30% vs. 51%), with an absolute risk reduction of 21% (95% CI, 3–38%) and an unadjusted odds ratio of 0.41 (95% CI, 0.180.89; $P = 0.03$). The median numbers of days free of invasive ventilation within 28 days from enrollment were 28 (IQR, 13–28) in the helmet group vs. 25 (IQR, 4–28) in the HFNO group, a difference that was statistically significant (95% CI, 0–7; $P = 0.04$) [5].

Other advantages in the use of the helmet are: superior mask seal (especially in patients with facial hair or unusual anatomy), reduced aspiration risk, reduced risk of skin injuries, and no requirement of mechanical ventilator (e.g., can be run directly off wall oxygen). To conclude, face-mask NIV generated conflicting results, while Helmet NIV demonstrated a good tolerability, improved oxygenation, and prevented lung injury [5].

12.3 Ventilation-Related Risks and Contraindications

The greatest concerns related to the application of NIV in COVID-19 AHRF are the risk of patient self-inflicted lung injury (P-SILI), delayed intubation, and the spread of the virus in the environment [6].

As well-known, non-invasive respiratory support cannot guarantee lung protective ventilation: severely hypoxemic patients usually exhibit high respiratory drive and vigorous efforts that enhance P-SILI through tidal volume increase, pendelluft phenomenon, capillary leak, lung edema, and excessive intrathoracic negative pressures. In addition, despite fully fitting the ARDS Berlin definition, the discrepancies between the severity of oxygenation impairment, the characteristics of lung mechanics, and the atypical lung CT-imaging raises the hypothesis that the underlying pathophysiology of COVID-19-induced ARDS (CARDS) is fundamentally different from the typical ARDS. These characteristics are particularly observed during the early clinical stages, when the perfusion dysregulation is more clinically significant than lung edema or atelectasis. According to Gattinoni, in the early CARDS pneumonia (type L phenotype), high PEEP or CPAP may be useless or even harmful, with hemodynamic impairment and fluid retention as a consequence of the rise of total lung stress, which seems to be the only variable independently associated with NIV failure and intubation. However, it is still questionable if a high stress contributes to worsening of COVID-19 pneumonia or if the worsening of pneumonia contributes to an increased stress, so further research is needed [7, 8].

Given the high probability of failure (up to 50% in various studies), NIV-treated patients should be hospitalized in an ICU environment where more efficient resource allocation and continuous monitoring can be established [9]. Nevertheless, in the context of the COVID-19 pandemic, there is a huge need to use non-invasive modes of ventilation outside the ICU in order to spare ICU beds [6]. During the first COVID-19 wave in Italy, a "feasibility study" established that non-invasive respiratory support can be successfully applied outside an ICU; subsequently plenty of studies from different countries described successful application of CPAP or NIV in many wards with the vast majority of patients receiving CPAP support [10].

However, there is no consensus on the optimal timing of CPAP/NIV application in patients affected by AHRF associated with Sars-Cov-2 infection. Particularly in non-ICU settings, close monitoring and continuous evaluation of predictors of failure are essential in order not to delay invasive mechanical ventilation in patients who are not responding to the treatment within the first 1–2 h [1, 11].

Many researches evidenced that PaO2 / FiO2 < 150 mmHg, expiratory tidal volume > 9.5 mL/kg PBW, and HACOR score (heart rate, pH, Glasgow coma scale, PaO2/FiO2 and respiratory rate) > 5 at 1 h of NIV carry a high probability of failure [6, 12–16]. According to these findings, Ward-COVID, the largest multicenter study from Italy, demonstrated NIV failure in 53% of patients with PaO2 /FiO2 < 150 mmHg vs. 18% in patients with PaO2/FiO2 > 150 mmHg; Coppadoro et al. likewise showed that PaO2/ FiO2 < 100 mmHg with helmet CPAP was associated with a higher risk of failure [17, 18]. In addition, Menga et al. claimed that independent factors associated with non-invasive oxygen support failure were SAPS II score ($P = 0.009$) and serum lactate dehydrogenase at enrollment ($P = 0.02$); the combination of SAPS II score ≥ 33 with serum LDH ≥ 405 units/L at ICU admission had 91% specificity in predicting the need for tracheal intubation [19].

On the other hand, an increase in oxygenation with CPAP treatment and a decrease in the respiratory rate (<24/min) were strong indices of success [18].

National and international guidelines (WHO, 2020; CCCGWG, 2020; NCCET, 2020; Indian CDC, 2020; NHS (NIV), 2020; ICSI, 2020) suggest that patients with worsening respiratory status or lack of improvement despite NIV support within 1–2 h (PaO2/FiO2 < 100 mmHg), development of respiratory acidosis–hypercapnia (PaCO2 > 45 mmHg with pH < 7.35), higher risk of regurgitation or aspiration, severe facial skin injuries, hemodynamic instability, sepsis or multiorgan dysfunction (SOFA > 4), and abnormal mental status should not receive NIV and tracheal intubation should not be delayed [4].

12.4 Contamination-Related Hazard and Practical Recommendations for Hospital Management

The potential increased risk of healthcare personnel contamination related to management of COVID-19 patients with non-invasive respiratory modalities is still debated. Simulation or observational studies conducted before the COVID-19 pandemic are substantially inconclusive.

Undoubtedly, environmental contamination is higher in patients treated with these modalities compared to mechanical ventilation with closed suction systems, but there is no significant difference in the risk of aerosol production and dispersion between them and spontaneous breathing or conventional oxygen treatment. Moreover, the infection control efficacy of many mask/filter units has not been well evaluated. Factors such as augmented positive pressures during NIV and poor fit of these devices to the patient's face carry a higher risk of viral transmission [6, 20–23]. In December 2020, Canadian Anesthesiologists' Society affirmed that the use of CPAP/NIV may increase the risk of mistakes in donning PPE due to time pressures to resuscitate or intubate in emergency situations [24].

International institutions recommend to take appropriate precautions to reduce any hazard: negative-pressure or dedicated confirmed-cases wards; hand hygiene; personal protective equipment, including N95 or higher respirators, eye protection, gloves and long-sleeved, water-repellent single-use coat; well-fitted devices with no leaks; positive pressures and flow rates at the minimum necessary [3, 4]. Moreover, the better tolerability of the helmet and reduced room contamination might also improve both clinical management of patients and the safety of the healthcare workers [25]. When helmet NIV cannot be used, Hudson and Venturi masks or a face mask combined with a double circuit with an expiratory valve and an antimicrobial and antiviral filter might be suggested (ITS & IRS, 2020) [4].

Several studies demonstrated no disease transmission to healthcare workers from patients treated with NIV if they follow the mentioned appropriate personal protection precautions and nosocomial strategies [3].

References

1. Clinical management of severe acute respiratory infection when novel coronavirus infection is suspected. WHO Interim Guidance, 12 january 2020.
2. Carter C, Aedy H, Notter J. COVID-19 disease: non-invasive ventilation and high frequency nasal oxygenation. Clinics Integr Care. 2020;1:100006.
3. Jeschke KN, Bonnesen B, Hansen EF, Jensen J-US, Lapperre TS, Weinreich UM, Hilberg O. Guideline for the management of COVID-19 patients during hospital admission in a non-intensive care setting. Eur Clin Respir J. 2020;7(1):1761677.
4. Wang Z, et al. The use of non-invasive ventilation in COVID-19: a systematic review. Int J Infect Dis. 2021;106:254–61.
5. Grieco DL, Menga LS, Cesarano M, et al. Helmet vs HFNO NIV in COVID-19 gemelli IRCS. JAMA. 2021;325(17):1731–43.
6. Akoumianaki E, Ischaki E, Karagiannis K, Sigala I, Zakyn-thinos S. The role of noninvasive respiratory management in patients with severe COVID-19 pneumonia. J Pers Med. 2021;11:884.
7. Gattinoni L, Coppola S, et al. Role of total lung stress on the progression of early COVID-19 pneumonia. Intensive Care Med. 2021;47:1130–9.
8. Gattinoni L, et al. COVID-19 pneumonia: different respiratory treatment for different phenotypes? Intensive Care Med. 2020;46(6):1099–102.
9. Grieco DL, Menga LS, Cesarano M, Rosà T, Spadaro S, Bitondo MM, Montomoli J, Falò G, Tonetti T, Cutuli SL, et al. Effect of helmet noninvasive ventilation versus high-flow nasal oxygen on days free

of respiratory support in patients with COVID-19 and moderate to severe hypoxemic respiratory failure: the HENIVOT randomized clinical trial. JAMA. 2021;325:1731.

10. Franco C, Facciolongo N, Tonelli R, Dongilli R, Vianello A, Pisani L, Scala R, Malerba M, Carlucci A, Negri EA, et al. Feasibility and clinical impact of out-of-ICU noninvasive respiratory support in patients with COVID-19-related pneumonia. Eur Respir J. 2020;56:2002130.

11. Chalmers JD, Crichton ML, Goeminne PC, et al. Management of hospitalised adults with coronavirus disease 2019 (COVID-19): a European respiratory society living guideline. Eur Respir J. 2021;57:2100048.

12. Alviset S, Riller Q, Aboab J, et al. Continuous positive airway pressure (CPAP) face-mask ventilation is an easy and cheap option to manage a massive influx of patients presenting acute respiratory failure during the SARS-CoV-2 outbreak: a retrospective cohort study. PLoS One. 2020;15:e0240645.

13. Carteaux G, Millán-Guilarte T, De Prost N, et al. A failure of noninvasive ventilation for de novo acute hypoxemic respiratory failure: role of tidal volume. Crit Care Med. 2016;44:282–90.

14. Frat JP, Ragot S, Coudroy R, et al. Predictors of intubation in patients with acute hypoxemic respiratory failure treated with a noninvasive oxygenation strategy. Crit Care Med. 2018;46:208–15.

15. Carrillo A, Lopez A, Carrillo L, et al. Validity of a clinical scale in predicting the failure of non-invasive ventilation in hypoxemic patients. J Crit Care. 2020;60:152–8.

16. Duan J, Han X, Bai L, Zhou L, Huang S. Assessment of heart rate, acidosis, consciousness, oxygenation, and respiratory rate to predict noninvasive ventilation failure in hypoxemic patients. Intensive Care Med. 2017;43:192–9.

17. Bellani G, Grasselli G, Cecconi M, et al. Noninvasive ventilatory support of patients with COVID-19 outside the intensive care units (WARd-COVID). Ann ATS. 2021;18:1020–6.

18. Coppadoro A, Benini A, Fruscio R, et al. Helmet CPAP to treat hypoxic pneumonia outside the ICU: an observational study during the COVID-19 outbreak. Crit Care. 2021;25:80.

19. Menga LS, Cese LD, Bongiovanni F, Lombardi G, Michi T, Luciani F, Cicetti M, Timpano J, Ferrante MC, Cesarano M, et al. High failure rate of noninvasive oxygenation strategies in critically ill subjects with acute hypoxemic respiratory failure due to COVID-19. Respir Care. 2021;66:705–14.

20. Gaeckle NT, Lee J, Park Y, et al. Aerosol generation from the respiratory tract with various modes of oxygen delivery. Am J Respir Crit Care Med. 2020;202:1115–24.

21. Iwashyna TJ, Boehman A, Capecelatro J, et al. Variation in aerosol production across oxygen delivery devices in spontaneously breathing human subjects. medRxiv. 2020:20066688.

22. Miller DC, Beamer P, Billheimer D, et al. Aerosol risk with noninvasive respiratory support in patients with COVID-19. J Am Coll Emerg Physicians Open. 2020;1:521–6.

23. Hui DS, Chow BK, Lo T, et al. Exhaled air dispersion during high-flow nasal cannula therapy versus CPAP via different masks. Eur Respir J. 2019;53:1802339.

24. Wax RS, Christian MD. Practical recommendations for critical care and anesthesiology teams caring for novel coronavirus (2019-nCoV) patients. Can J Anesth/J Can Anesth. 2020;67:568–76.

25. Radovanovic D, Rizzi M, Pini S, Saad M, Chiumello DA, Santus P. Helmet CPAP to treat acute hypoxemic respiratory failure in patients with COVID-19: a management strategy proposal. J Clin Med. 2020;9(4):1191.

Carmine Iacovazzo, Claudia Veropalumbo,
Maria Vargas, and Giuseppe Servillo

Contents

13.1 Introduction

Non-invasive ventilation (NIV) use in emergency departments and intensive care units (ICUs) increased in recent times. The major indications for its use are Acute Respiratory Failure (ARF) in patients with chronic obstructive pulmonary disease, acute cardiogenic pulmonary edema, and post-extubation respiratory failure, [1] but there is a spreading interest for its value in trauma patients, and lately various systematic reviews and meta-analyses have been published [2–4].

13.2 Acute Respiratory Failure in Trauma

Injury and trauma persist to be the number one cause of death in U.S. and E.U. citizens aged 1–44 [5, 6]. Deaths directly related to severe trauma often occur within hours of injury, even before hospitalization and trauma victims who

C. Iacovazzo · C. Veropalumbo (✉) · M. Vargas ·
G. Servillo
Department of Neuroscience and Reproductive and
Odontostomatological Sciences, Intensive Care Unit,
University of Naples Federico II, Naples, Italy
e-mail: giuseppe.servillo@unina.it

© The Author(s), under exclusive license to Springer Nature Switzerland AG 2023
G. Servillo, M. Vargas (eds.), *Non-invasive Mechanical Ventilation in Critical Care, Anesthesiology
and Palliative Care*, https://doi.org/10.1007/978-3-031-36510-2_13

survive their initial injuries to hospitalization cope with the risk of life-threatening complications such as Multiple Organ Failure (MOF), [7–9] the major cause of death in these patients [10]. The most frequent manifestation of MOF after trauma is acute respiratory distress syndrome (ARDS); [11] therefore, acute respiratory failure (ARF) represents a primary challenge in the management of trauma, affecting up to 20% of complex trauma patients [12, 13]. Injured patients with ARDS and MOF present mortality rates from 50% to 80% [11, 14].

13.3 Pathophysiology of Acute Respiratory Failure in Trauma

Acute respiratory failure following trauma can be the consequence of direct chest injury, inducing a functional impairment of one or both lungs, as well as indirect injury via a multifactorial inflammatory-mediated response to severe extra-thoracic injury.

13.4 Direct Chest Trauma

13.4.1 Blunt Thoracic Trauma

The most frequent injury found in blunt thoracic trauma is *pulmonary contusion*, which may lead to ARF through a multitude of pathophysiologic changes, such as alterations in surfactant stabilization of alveolar units, increased production of mucus and decreased clearance of mucus and blood from the airways, alterations of lung compliance, and ventilation/perfusion mismatch [15]. Pulmonary contusion promotes the development of acute lung injury (ALI), which may progress to acute respiratory distress syndrome (ARDS).

Frequently associated with pulmonary contusion, the presence of *rib fractures* may lead to ARF as a consequence of impairment in the cohesive function of the chest wall as a unit capable of granting negative pressure and providing full lung expansion, especially if in presence of severe pain; consequently, rib fractures predispose to significant *atelectasis*.

Furthermore, a *flail chest* occurs when a segment of the chest wall does not have bony continuity with the rest of the thoracic cage, as a result of the fracture of three or more ribs in two places or when there are multiple fractures associated with sternal fracture. The ARF associated with flail chest has been shown to be due to the underlying pulmonary contusion rather than paradoxical respiration [16].

Atelectasis causes ventilation-perfusion mismatch and hypoxemia refractory to supplemental oxygen and interferes with the clearance of bacteria, such as Streptococcus Pneumoniae, Staphylococcus Aureus, and Klebsiella Pneumoniae, which are frequent pathogens in early post-traumatic pneumonia [17, 18].

13.4.2 Penetrating Chest Trauma

Like blunt injury, penetrating thoracic injury can induce respiratory failure. In addition to the systemic inflammatory-mediated respiratory failure observed in severe injuries to other compartments, penetrating thoracic injury causes ARF by affecting lung parenchyma directly.

13.4.3 Pneumothorax

Injuries of the lungs or the thoracic wall can create a pleural injury, leading to the collection of air in the pleural space, which causes the collapse of the lung. Consequently, all penetrating thoracic injuries and most blunt chest injuries are associated with pneumothorax. Occult pneumothorax among victims of blunt trauma appears in 2–55% of patients who undergo CT scans [19], therefore chest radiograph or CT scan should be the initial test for all patients with penetrating chest injuries [20] or blunt thoracic trauma; [21] ultrasound may also be useful in the diagnosis of pneumothorax, [22] whose presence is mandatory to be excluded before starting positive pressure ventilation. Patients affected by pneumothorax who needs to be mechanically ventilated should be treated immediately with a tube thoracostomy to prevent the development of tension pneumothorax.

13.5 Indirect Chest Trauma

Aside from direct traumatic injury to the thorax, severe extrathoracic injury can also cause respiratory failure through a variety of mechanisms.

Traumatic brain injury (TBI) has a close link with respiratory failure, and approximately 1/3 of severe TBI patients manifest it [23]. ARF from TBI can be the result of impaired respiratory drive due to neural injury, but also TBI lead to increased endothelial permeability at both the blood-brain and the blood-lung barriers; [24, 25] furthermore, elevated intracranial pressure has been shown to induce pulmonary edema [26].

In addition, fat embolism from long bone fractures [27] and venous thrombosis complicating major trauma [28] can lead to lung injury and ARF, sometimes even in the immediate post-injury setting.

Moreover, severely injured trauma patients frequently require blood products transfusion: it doubles the risk for the onset and evolution of acute lung injury in the 6–72 h after the transfusion [29, 30].

13.6 Ventilatory Management

When ARF occurs, respiratory support in the presence of both direct and indirect traumatic lung injury shares the same management goals: maintain lung recruitment and gas exchange, while avoiding ventilator-associated lung injury (VALI).

13.7 Definitive Airway

According to Advanced Trauma Life Support (ATLS) protocol [31], the criteria for establishing a definitive airway (orotracheal/nasotracheal tube, cricothyroidotomy, or tracheostomy) are based on clinical signs and include:

- Inability to maintain a patent airway with other aids, with oncoming or potential airway compromise (e.g., following inhalation injury, facial fractures, or retropharyngeal hematoma);
- Presence of apnea;
- Inability to maintain adequate oxygenation by facemask oxygen supplementation;
- Obtundation or combativeness caused by cerebral hypoperfusion;
- Presence of a head injury with severe neurologic impairment (Glasgow Coma Scale score of 8 or less) or sustained seizure activity, and the subsequent need to protect the lower airway from aspiration of blood or vomitus.

Notoriously, endotracheal intubation (ETI), especially in patients with pulmonary contusion, is associated with the risk of developing ventilator-associated pneumonia (VAP) [32] and increased incidence of pneumonia in intubated chest and abdominal trauma patients has been demonstrated; thus, invasive mechanical ventilation could add another risk factor for pulmonary complications, therefore when gas exchange is not too severely compromised and when there are no contraindications to non-invasive positive pressure ventilation (NIPPV), tracheal intubation should be avoided.

13.8 Non-invasive Ventilation

In selected patients with no contraindications to NIPPV/indications to ETI, Non-Invasive Ventilation (NIV) could be the winning strategy of respiratory support.

Concerning the possible clinical applications of NIPPV in trauma patients with ARF, it may be used beginning with out-of-hospital first aid settings [33] and in the emergency settings. As already mentioned, the possible presence of a pneumothorax must be excluded in the first place or treated by a chest drainage.

In the ICU, patients may be treated by NIV in order to reduce the need for intubation [34]. Moreover, even if the patient needs ETI, early extubation (when possible) and maintenance of gas exchange by NIV prevent the onset of invasive mechanical ventilation-related pulmonary complications [35].

In major trauma patients, a ventilation strategy that minimizes airway pressure and ensures permissive hypercapnia is of great concern, meaning that the strategy of *protective mechanical ventilation* should be applied by reducing lung distension and preventing end-expiratory collapse [36].

The practice of setting *tidal volumes of 6 mL/kg* of predicted body weight and limiting the plateau pressure ($P_{plat} < 28$–30 cm H_2O) has now been universally accepted in patients with ARDS [37, 38]. This minimization in tidal volume may lead to alveolar decruitment if not enough positive end-expiratory pressure (PEEP) is applied: the use of high PEEP may result in excessive lung parenchyma stress and strain [39] and this may have a more severe impact on a yet compromised lung.

The level of PEEP used to prevent alveolar collapse has been studied in a systematic review and meta-analysis [40]: the practice of a *high PEEP strategy*, despite a possible increased risk of biotrauma, seems to be the winning strategy. PEEP should be incrementally added to optimize gas exchange and may reach a range of 14–16 cm H_2O in patients with severe lung injury [41]. However, severe hypotension and a meaningful reduction of cardiac output have to be avoided.

Elevated $PaCO_2$ levels can be tolerated (*permissive hypercapnia*) for level of pH higher than 7.2, except in patients with elevated intracranial pressures.

FiO_2 should be as low as possible: unsettled initial situations in traumatized patients require high FiO_2 values, but under controlled conditions of an ICU, FIO_2 should be adapted to obtain oxygen saturation $\geq 90\%$.

With regard to the method of NIPPV administration, unfortunately, scientific literature is still scant of evidence that can be used in the choice of the best mode of ventilation.

The avoidance of airway and alveolar collapse granted by Continuous Positive Airway Pressure (CPAP) prevents atelectasis, maintains functional residual capacity, and reduces inspiratory muscle work and, at the same time, alleviates patient's pain, but in patients with pulmonary contusion, ventilation modalities such as bi-level or PSV have now become much more common than CPAP, even if superiority is not been demonstrated [42].

Otherwise in patients with flail chest injury, some findings suggest that CPAP provides more effective pneumatic stabilization than any other positive pressure ventilation, which may allow for fibrous chest wall stability and recovery [43].

As a matter of fact, the improvement in the outcome that may be obtained with NIV is not devoid of side effects: positive pressure ventilation can raise intracranial pressure and consequently decrease cerebral perfusion pressure, which can be of concern in TBI. Moreover, the increased intrathoracic pressure compromises venous return which, in addition to the consequence of the fluid restriction, is largely applied to patients with lung injury.

13.9 Conclusion

The attention to the role of NIV in trauma settings is reasonably growing, even if in 2002 the British Thoracic Society Standards of Care Committee gave only a grade C recommendation on the use of NIV for patients with chest wall trauma because of lack of evidence [44]. However, since then there have been several studies looking specifically at the use of NIV in traumatic patients and systematic reviews and meta-analysis about this topic were recently published. Unfortunately, as remarked by Duggal et al., [45] there is a great clinical heterogeneity among studies: if NIV is compared with all other strategies, it shows a protective effect, but this effect is poor if we examine only RCT, [2] although with still shorter ICU and hospital length of stay.

NIV appears to be safe and improves outcomes when used in appropriately selected patients; however, strong evidence is still lacking and consequently there is no uniform consensus among different societies to recommend use of NIV in trauma patients. Only an increased application and a greater diffusion could lead to achieve the required investigation in order to better define the role of NIV in the trauma population.

References

1. Ferrer M, Torres A. Noninvasive ventilation for acute respiratory failure. Curr Opin Crit Care. 2015;21:1–6.
2. Chiumello D, Coppola S, Froio S, et al. Noninvasive ventilation in chest trauma: systematic review and meta-analysis. Intensive Care Med. 2013;39:1171–80.
3. Duggal A, Perez P, Golan E, et al. Safety and efficacy of noninvasive ventilation in patients with blunt chest trauma: a systematic review. Crit Care. 2013;17:R142.
4. Roberts S, Skinner D, Biccard B, Rodseth RN. The role of non-invasive ventilation in blunt chest trauma: systematic review and meta-analysis. Eur J Trauma Emerg Surg. 2014;40:553–9.
5. Centers for Disease Control and Prevention. Web-based injury statistics query and reporting system (WISQARS) [online] (1999–007). National Center for Injury Prevention and Control, Centers for Disease Control and Prevention; 2019.
6. Eurostat. Life expectancy by age and sex. 2022.
7. Acosta JA, Yang JC, Winchell RJ, et al. Lethal injuries and time to death in a level I trauma center. 1998. J Am Coll Surg. 1998;186:528–33.
8. Sauaia A, Moore FA, Moore EE, et al. Epidemiology of trauma deaths: a reassessment. J Trauma. 1995;38:185–93.
9. Stewart RM, Myers JG, Dent DL, et al. Seven hundred fifty-three consecutive deaths in a level I trauma center: the argument for injury prevention. J Trauma. 2003;54(1):66–70.
10. Marshall JC, Cook DJ, Christou NV, et al. Multiple organ dysfunction score: a reliable descriptor of a complex clinical outcome. Crit Care Med. 1995;23(10):1638–52. 1992, Vol. 23, pp. 1638–1652.
11. Sauaia A, Moore FA, Moore EE, et al. Early predictors of postinjury multiple organ failure. Arch Surg. 1994;129(1):39–45.
12. Geiger EV, Lustenberger T, Wutzler S, et al. Predictors of pulmonary failure following severe trauma: a trauma registry-based analysis. Scand J Trauma Resusc Emerg Med. 2013;21:34.
13. Wutzler S, Wafaisade A, Maegele M, et al. Lung organ failure score (LOFS): probability of severe pulmonary organ failure after multiple injuries including chest trauma. Injury. 2012;43:1507–12.
14. Durham RM, Moran JJ, Mazuski JE, et al. Multiple organ failure in trauma patients. J Trauma. 2003;55:608–16.
15. Cohn SM, Dubose JJ. Pulmonary contusion: an update on recent advances in clinical management. World J Surg. 2010;34:1959–70.
16. Hurst JM, DeHaven CB, Branson RD. Use of CPAP mask as the sole mode of ventilatory support in trauma patients with mild to moderate respiratory insufficiency. J Trauma. 1985;25:1065–8.
17. van Kaam AH, Lachmann RA, Herting E, et al. Reducing atelectasis attenuates bacterial growth and translocation in experimental pneumonia. Am J Respir Crit Care Med. 2004;169(9):1046–53.
18. Croce MA, Fabian TC, Mueller EW, Maish GO, et al. The appropriate diagnostic threshold for ventilator-associated pneumonia using quantitative cultures. J Trauma. 2004;56:931–6.
19. Ball CG, Kirkpatrick AW, Laupland KB, Fox DI, Nicolaou S, Anderson IB, et al. Incidence, risk factors, and outcomes for occult pneumothoraces in victims of major trauma. J Trauma. 2005;59:917–24.
20. Bokhari F, Brakenridge S, Nagy K, Roberts R, Smith R, Joseph K, et al. Prospective evaluation of the sensitivity of physical examination in chest trauma. J Trauma. 2002;53:1135–8.
21. Ho ML, Gutierrez FR. Chest radiography in thoracic polytrauma, vol. 192. AJR Am J Roentgenol; 2009. p. 599–612.
22. Dulchavsky SA, Hamilton DR, Diebel LN, Sargsyan AE, Billica RD, Williams DR. Thoracic ultrasound diagnosis of pneumothorax. J Trauma. 1999;47:970–1.
23. Pelosi P, Severgnini P, Chiaranda M. An integrated approach to prevent and treat respiratory failure in brain-injured patients. Curr Opin Crit Care. 2005;11:37–42.
24. Yildirim E, Solaroglu I, Okutan O, et al. Ultrastructural changes in tracheobronchial epithelia following experimental traumatic brain injury in rats: protective effect of erythropoietin. J Heart Lung Transplant. 2004;23:1423–9.
25. Rhodes JK, Andrews PJ, Holmes MC, et al. Expression of interleukin-6 messenger RNA in a rat model of diffuse axonal injury. Neurosci Lett. 2002;335(s.l):1–4.
26. AB, Malik. Mechanisms of neurogenic pulmonary edema. Circ Res. 1985;57:1–18.
27. Meyer N, Pennington WT, Dewitt D, et al. Isolated cerebral fat emboli syndrome in multiply injured patients: a review of three cases and the literature. J Trauma. 2007;63:1395–402.
28. Spencer Netto F, Tien H, Ng J, et al. Pulmonary emboli after blunt trauma: timing, clinical characteristics and natural history. Injury. 2012;43:1502–6.
29. Chaiwat O, Lang JD, Vavilala MS, et al. Early packed red blood cell transfusion and acute respiratory distress syndrome after trauma. Anesthesiology. 2009;110:351–60.
30. Watson GA, Sperry JL, Rosengart MR, et al. Fresh frozen plasma is independently associated with a higher risk of multiple organ failure and acute respiratory distress syndrome. J Trauma. 2009;67:221–30.
31. American College of Surgeons. ATLS-advanced trauma life support. Chicago: Committee on Trauma; 2018.

32. Antonelli M, Moro ML, Capelli O, et al. Risk factors for early onset pneumonia in trauma patients. Chest. 1994;105:224–8.

33. Pandor A, Thokala P, Goodacre S, et al. Pre-hospital non-invasive ventilation for acute respiratory failure: a systematic review and cost-effectiveness evaluation. Health Technol Assess. 2015;19:1–102.

34. Beltrame F, Lucangelo U, Gregori D, Gregoretti C. Noninvasive positive pressure ventilation in trauma patients with acute respiratory failure. Monaldi Arch Chest Dis. 1999;54:109–14.

35. Gregoretti C, Beltrame F, Lucangelo U, et al. Physiologic evaluation of non-invasive pressure support ventilation in trauma patients with acute respiratory failure. Intensive Care Med. 1998;24:785–90.

36. Richter T, Ragaller M. Ventilation in chest trauma. J Emerg Trauma Shock. 2011;4(2):251–9.

37. Amato MD, Barbas CS, Medeiros DM, et al. Effect of protective-ventilation strategy on mortality in acute respiratory distress syndrome. N Engl J Med. 1998;338:347–54.

38. Meade MO, Cook DJ, Guyatt GH, et al. Ventilation strategy using low tidal volumes, recruitment maneuvers, and high positive end-expiratory pressure for acute lung injury and acute respiratory distress syndrome: randomized control trial. JAMA. 2008;229:637–45.

39. Imai Y, Paroda J, Kajikawa O, et al. Injurious mechanical ventilation and endorgan epithelial cell apoptosis and organ dysfunction in an experimental model of acute respiratory distress. JAMA. 2003;289:2104–12.

40. Phoenix SI, Paravastu S, Columb M, et al. Does a higher positive end expiratory pressure decrease mortality in acute respiratory distress syndrome? Anesthesiology. 2009;110:1098–105.

41. Papadakos PJ, Karcz M, Lachmann B. Mechanical ventilation in trauma. Curr Opin Anaesthesiol. 2010;23:228–32.

42. Xirouchaki N, Kondoudaki E, Anastasaki M, et al. Noninvasive bilevel positive pressure ventilation in patients with blunt thoracic trauma. Respiration. 2005;72:517–22.

43. Pettiford L, Luketich JD, Landreneau RJ. The Management of Flail Chest. Thorac Surg Clin. 2007;17:25–33.

44. Committee, British Thoracic Society Standard of Care. Non-invasive ventilation in acute respiratory failure. Thorax. 2002;57:192–211.

45. Hernandez G, Fernandez R, Lopez-Reina P, et al. Noninvasive ventilation reduces intubation in chest trauma-related hypoxemia. Chest. 2010;137:74–80.

Non-invasive Ventilation in Post-extubation Failure

Marco Rispoli and Maurizia Lanza

Contents

14.1 The Importance of Extubation and Its Relevance in ICU Patients

Mechanical ventilation is a life-saving procedure, but it is not risk-free, especially if keeping over time because mortality increases with duration of intubation and so do other complications related to mechanical ventilation such as upper airway lesions, prolonged immobility, mechanical injury to lung parenchyma, and infections associated or not with ventilator. In addition to the prevention of complications, the removal of the endotracheal tube entails a series of advantages for the comfort of the patient, improving communication, reducing the need for sedation, ensuring an effective cough and, where possible, return to normal diet. Traditionally, clinicians have always stressed the need to make the patient "free" from the mechanical ventilator, switching the work of breathing from machine to man, in order to minimize his dependence on such external support. The crucial importance of this manoeuvre is underlined by the fact that up to 40–60% of mechanical ventilation time is spent weaning the patient. Usually, at the end of such weaning procedure, the patient is automatically considered to no longer need the endotracheal tube and is ready for the extubation. This is not always true and, in case of extubation-

M. Rispoli (✉)
Department of Critical Care, Anesthesia and Intensive Care, AO dei Colli, Monaldi Hospital, Naples, Italy

M. Lanza
Department of Critical Care, Respiratory Physiopathology, AO dei Colli, Monaldi Hospital, Naples, Italy

© The Author(s), under exclusive license to Springer Nature Switzerland AG 2023
G. Servillo, M. Vargas (eds.), *Non-invasive Mechanical Ventilation in Critical Care, Anesthesiology and Palliative Care*, https://doi.org/10.1007/978-3-031-36510-2_14

failure, there is a strong association with risk of prolonged mechanical ventilation, longer ICU stay, high mortality, and rise in cost of care. As shown by Coplin et al. [1], even a 48-h delay in extubation, once clinical stability has been achieved, leads to more pneumonia, longer stay in intensive care and hospital, and increased mortality.

Thus, clinicians are continuously balancing the need to extubate promptly their patients against the risk of extubation failure with its consequent impact on outcomes.

14.1.1 Extubation Failure, an Underestimated Problem

"if you never re-intubate your patient in an emergency, it means you do not extubate enough" Owens [2] jokingly said in his ventilator book, and indeed the magnitude of the problem ranges from 2% to 25%. This wide prevalence gap depends on the non-constant definition of failed extubation in the medical literature (24 h, 72 h or even a week). The context in which extubation takes place also plays a specific role: in fact, in the operating theatres all over the world, many extubations are performed but, in the case of the surgical patient to be extubated at the end of the intervention, failure is recorded only in 5% of cases (including trauma and cardiothoracic surgery). Some factors determine a greater frequency of problems with extubation: medical, pediatric, and multi-pathology patients hospitalized in the ICU are more exposed. Another risk factor is the physicians-patient and nurses-patient ratio, especially during night shifts. Specifically, Dang et al. [3] and Amaravadi et al. [4] demonstrated that a nurse-to-patient ratio of less than 1:2 resulted in a higher incidence of reintubation in abdominal aortic and esophagus surgery.

The most common risk factors are:

- Older age (>65 years)
- COPD
- Congestive heart
- Pneumonia
- High severity of illness
- Prolonged immobility
- Mechanical ventilation >7 days
- Positive fluid balance prior to extubation
- Ineffective cough
- Abundant respiratory secretions
- Abnormal mental status, delirium
- Upper airway obstruction
- Rapid shallow breathing
- Hypercapnia at the conclusion of a SBT or immediately after extubation
- Post-extubation dysphagia
- Morbid obesity

The increased need for ICU following failed extubation ranges from prolonged mechanical ventilation (up to 12 days), extended ICU stay (up to 21 days), and prolonged hospitalization up to 30 days. Furthermore, failure of extubation, especially if repeated, is a risk factor for tracheostomy. Pronovost et al. [5] estimated that these consequences of extubation failure can increase patient management costs by 20%, adding a cost-effectiveness aspect to the management of this problem.

In addition to increased complications and length of hospitalization, patients experiencing failed extubation have a higher mortality that ranges from 2 to 10 times that of uncomplicated extubated patients in univariate studies [6]. But, even in multivariate analysis—considering the different comorbidities and severity of illness—an independent association with mortality is reported. The only condition in which this association with mortality is less marked is in cases of extubation failure due to lack of airway patency or inadequate secretion clearance compared to respiratory or heart failure.

The motivation for this strong association between re-intubation and mortality is still unclear. One possibility is that mortality is related to the stress and complications that the tracheal intubation manoeuvre itself entails.

Another theory is that the extubation failure may depend on the worsening of the underlying clinical status.

Another hypothesis is related to the lack of ventilatory support during post-extubation observation: the longer the elapsed time between extubation and eventual reintubation, the higher the incidence of complications. In fact, extubation failure is defined by the presence of at least two of the following signs of distress:

- Hypercapnia (PaCO2 > 45 mmHg or > 20% increase from pre-extubation)
- Respiratory acidosis (pH < 7.35 with PaCO2 > 45 mmHg)
- Clinical signs of respiratory muscle fatigue or increased work of breathing
- Respiratory rate (RR) of >25 breaths/min for two consecutive hours
- Hypoxaemia (SpO2 < 90% or PaO2 < 80 mmHg on FiO2 > 0.50)

Such distress conditions, especially if continued for hours, can severely impact the patient's status. Supporting this hypothesis is the evidence shown by De Lassence et al. [7] in which no increase in mortality is reported in case of accidental extubation with immediate re-intubation (within a maximum of 1 h). Therefore, it would not seem to be the failure of extubation itself, but the ability to provide immediate ventilator support to the patient, the likely cause of mortality.

This leads us to underline how prevention of failed extubation can allow us to anticipate critical issues and reduce the time of exposure to an inadequate ventilation support of our patient.

14.2 Physiology of Extubation Failure and Its Prevention

Commonly, patients fail at managing the spontaneous work of breathe due to fatigue. In fact, patients not tolerating spontaneous breathing test manifest high respiratory rate with shallow breathing, increased elastic and resistive work of breathing, rise in intrinsic PEEP, deficit of gas exchange, respiratory muscle exhaustion, and increased tension–time index (inspiratory time over the total breath duration).

For these reasons, the possibility to prevent an extubation failure may rely on the common ventilation parameters even if most of medical literature agree that they have a limited utility:

- Vital capacity
- Minute ventilation
- Respiratory rate
- Tidal volume
- Negative inspiratory force
- Maximal inspiratory pressure
- Work of breathing

Considering more sophisticated measurements, one of the most widespread and well-studied tests is the Respiratory Rate/Tidal volume ratio. In this test, the ratio between high respiratory frequency and the low tidal volume of patients not tolerating the spontaneous breathing will be higher with a cut-off for extubation failure of 105. But even this parameter rarely leads to moderate or large changes in the probability of success or failure. The study of the breathing pattern during spontaneous breathing trial may predict extubation failure, also gas exchange analysis and the presence of elevated volume of dead space (volume of dead space/tidal volume > 0.65) may relate to extubation failure. McCool et al. [8] used ultrasound measures of diaphragm thickness or diaphragm dome excursion to predict extubation success or failure, while Ferrè et al. [9] used lung ultrasound score to detect weaning-induced pulmonary edema.

Airway patency must be satisfactory before attempting an extubation because, in case of upper airway obstruction, the work of breathe could increase and force to re-intubate the patient after the endotracheal tube removal. A quantitative cuff leak test is usually performed to assess airway patency, as an indirect measurement of the volume of air leaking around the tube when the cuff is deflated. Unfortunately, despite a positive cuff leak test, an effective treatment is still not available to reduce the upper airway obstruction. Anyway fewer than 50% of patients with stridor after extubation actually require reintubation and, also among those who need it, outcomes are much better compared to the ones re-intubated for respiratory or heart failure.

For what it concerns the proper airway protection during weaning, Bach and Saporito [10] studied patients with primarily neuromuscular causes for acute respiratory failure and reported that the extubation or decannulation failure be likely related with peak cough flow rates less than 160 L/min, while Duan et al. [11] reported a weak cough peak as predictor sign of extubation failure correlating the strength of cough with the respiratory muscle strength: patients with peak flow <70 L/min (measured connecting a spirometer to the endotracheal tube just before removal) needed more frequently NIV in the post-extubation phase because of respiratory distress.

Other risk factors for re-intubation due to lack of airway protection are:

- Presence of moderate to abundant secretions (patients requiring endotracheal suctioning more frequently than every 2 h)
- Brain dysfunction
- Depressed mental status

While there is no single perfect indicator to predict extubation failure, looking for signs of efficient work of breathing, airway patency, and protection is definitely a good approach. The ideal patient to extubate should easily pass the spontaneous breathing test and be able to count on a good cough in the absence of excessive secretions and without obstruction of the upper airways.

The most common pathophysiologic alterations after unsuccessful extubation are:

- Rapid shallow breathing
- Alterated gas exchange
- Reduced alveolar ventilation
- Increased work of breathing
- Intrinsic PEEP
- Dynamic hyperinflation
- Increased pulmonary artery pressure
- Abnormal left ventricular ejection fraction

In view of such pathological conditions, NIV appears to be the perfect answer being capable of reducing the work of breathing, improving oxygenation, and abolishing intrinsic PEEP granting reduction in respiratory rate and a better tidal volume.

14.3 Niv in Prevention of Post-extubation Respiratory Failure

Over time, it has become increasingly evident that the timing of application of NIV, after extubation, plays a fundamental role in its success.

Jiang et al. [12], among the first, hypothesized that early application of NIV after extubation, before respiratory decompensation, would reduce the incidence of extubation failure. While not finding any data to support the routine use of NIV, he reported that the rate of re-intubations was much higher among patients who had undergone accidental self-extubation (38%) compared to the planned one (11%), probably due to the lack of adequate preparation and correct timing. In a 406 patients RCT, Su et al. [13] used NIV to prevent re-intubation in unselected patients. Patients in the NIV group received 10–12 cm H_2O Pressure support and 5 cm H_2O PEEP. Support was increased according to pCO_2, while PEEP was raised to get $SpO_2 > 92\%$. The results of this study reported that NIV did not decrease extubation failure rate or ICU mortality. Therefore, the indiscriminate use of NIV does not seem to provide particular advantages in avoiding re-intubation.

A different approach was adopted by Nava et al. [14]; his group focused on patients with risk factors for extubation failure:

- More than one consecutive failure of weaning trial
- Chronic heart failure
- $PaCO_2 > 45$ mm Hg after extubation
- More than one comorbidity (excluding chronic heart failure)
- Weak cough
- Upper airways stridor at extubation not requiring immediate re-intubation

Forty-eight high-risk patients underwent NIV and 48 standard therapy. The NIV group was ventilated in pressure support at least 8 h a day for 48 h, aiming to: respiratory rate25 breaths/min, $SpO_2 > 92\%$, and pH > 7.35. After the first 48 h of NIV, every patient was assessed for possible ventilation withdrawn; otherwise ventilation went on. The results of this study were in counter-trend with those previously obtained; in fact, the NIV had reduced the rate of re-intubation and mortality in the ICU, stressing that—probably—NIV support should be used on high-risk patients. After few months, Ferrer et al. [15] in a RCT tested preventive NIV in patients at risk for extubation due to:

- Age > 65 years
- Cardiac failure as the cause of intubation
- APACHE II > 12 on the day of extubation

In the 79 patients of the non-invasive ventilation group, NIV was delivered for a period of 19 ± 8 h and the levels of inspiratory and expiratory positive airway pressure were 14 ± 2 and 5 ± 1 cm H_2O, respectively. In the NIV group, the incidence of respiratory failure post-extubation was reduced. In a subsequent paper, Ferrer et al. [16] conducted an RCT on 106 COPD patients with hypercapnia during the spontaneous breathing test compared to oxygen therapy alone. The rate of respiratory failure post-extubation was lower in the NIV group, but ICU and hospital mortality were similar, with a 90-day survival rate significantly improved in the NIV group.

The contrast of these results with the previous ones was explained by the authors: NIV was applied immediately and continuously applied after extubation, high proficiency in NIV use by the health care team, and a significantly higher proportion of COPD patients in the study (51%). The high presence of COPD patients in this RCT underlines how NIV can offer its maximum performance in patients at high risk with an underlying pathological condition NIV-responder.

This principle is the basis of the study of El-Solh et al. [17] who have applied preventive NIV in patients with BMI > 35 as severely obese patients are considered at high risk of developing respiratory complications. Sixty-eight obese patients received NIV immediately post-extubation for a minimum of 48 h on average for 16 h/day. Compared with controls, NIV was associated with decreased post-extubation respiratory failure (10% vs. 26%) and fewer re-intubations (10% vs. 21%). Anyway, the mortality was the same between the two groups.

In view of the current available evidence, NIV should be used to prevent post-extubation respiratory failure in high-risk patients, while its use is not recommended in non-high-risk patients.

14.4 Niv in Treatment of Post-extubation Respiratory Failure

Keenan et al. [18] first tested with a single centre RCT the use of NIV in post-extubation respiratory failure after several case series and case control studies. They compared NIV with standard oxygen treatment in 78 patients with tachypnoea and respiratory accessory muscles use, within 48 h of extubation.

Patient in NIV started with 4 cm H_2O PEEP and 9 cm H_2O support; in case of hypoxia, PEEP was raised 2 cm H_2O until $SpO_2 > 92\%$, while in case of hypercapnia support was increased of 2 cm H_2O until normal pH on arterial blood gas. At the end of the study, despite a trend toward a longer time to re-intubation in case of NIV, no differences in re-intubation rate, length of stay, and mortality were found in the two groups.

Esteban et al. [19] performed a large, multi-center, international study to determine if NIV would reduce the rate of death in ICU among 221 patients with post-extubation respiratory failure compared to standard therapy. Respiratory failure was identified by at least two of the following: respiratory acidosis, clinical signs suggestive of respiratory-muscle fatigue or increased respiratory effort, respiratory rate greater than 25 breaths per minute for two consecutive hours, hypoxemia ($SpO_2 < 90\%$).

NIV was set in pressure support, to achieve a tidal volume > 5 mL/kg and a respiratory rate < 25 breaths per minute. The FiO_2 and the PEEP were titrated to maintain the $SpO_2 > 90\%$.

The main result was that not only NIV did not reduce mortality or the need for re-intubation, but also the mortality rate tended to be higher among patients assigned to NIV (25% vs. 14%). Probably, the delay in re-intubation caused the increase in the risk of death in the NIV group (12.7 vs. 2.4 h). Authors concluded that NIV could be even harmful.

These results are confirmed by a meta-analysis from Lin et al. [20], reporting no benefit of NIV compared with standard treatment with respect to re-intubation rate and mortality.

There appears to be no advantage in using NIV for the treatment of post-extubation respiratory failure according to the RCTs; however, it should be noted that in these studies the percentage of COPD patients was low ($\approx 10\%$) and not all the participating centres had the same experience in NIV use. Probably, a more careful monitoring of patients with NIV and timely reintubation may avoid potential harm. However, the use of NIV is not currently recommended in the treatment of patients with established post-extubation respiratory failure. Girault et al. [21] involved 17 centres in an RCT with 208 patients with acute-on-chronic respiratory failure that compares—for patients who have failed the trial for extubation—the continuation of invasive ventilation, the administration of an NIV, or the traditional oxygen therapy. Re-intubation, complications, ICU stay, and hospital survival were the same between the three groups, though NIV reduced the weaning failure. Moreover, NIV was used as rescue therapy in 45% of patients who underwent invasive ventilation weaning and 57% patients who received oxygen; this may have narrowed the margin of difference in favour of the NIV. The results of these trials have prompted researchers to seek an application of NIV that exploits its benefits immediately for weaning and for prevention of extubation failure, in order to minimize the time lapse between respiratory failure and the use of NIV, a factor that seems to be decisive for the success of this technique.

14.5 Niv in Weaning Patients

One of the temptations that NIV offers is to remove the endotracheal tube as soon as possible to shorten the duration of mechanical ventilation.

For this reason, many authors have applied non-invasive support to their weaning strategies. The basic idea is to provide a non-invasive support that guarantees, on the one hand, adequate ventilation without the tube, and on the other, the safety of not having to provide an urgent intubation for the risk of extubation failure.

The first enthusiasms were born with some uncontrolled studies, such as that of Kilger et al. [22] that extubated 15 patients once they had satisfying gas exchange even if they had border line respiratory pattern (e.g.: Respiratory Rate ≤ 40 breaths/min and tidal volume ≥ 3 mL/kg). NIV was 15 cm H_2O pressure support and 5 cm H_2O PEEP after extubation for a median of 2 days. Thirteen of 15 patients were successfully extubated.

In a prospective study involving patient intubated due to acute hypercapnic respiratory failure, Vitacca et al. [23] assessed the physiological response to pressure support ventilation delivered before and after extubation. They demonstrated that:

- Patients' physiological response to pressure support is the same, with or without endotracheal tube
- The energy expenditures of the diaphragm are similar with the two modalities of pressure support
- With the same level of support, the minute ventilation was the same for both modes of ventilation
- Patients reported a more pronounced feeling of dyspnoea with invasive ventilation

The data from this study give a new push to the physiological rationale in NIV use as a weaning technique, providing evidence that it may fully substitute the traditional invasive mechanical ventilation. Based on this physiological rationale, NIV has been increasingly used as a means to speed up the weaning process and to avoid the side effects and complications of endotracheal intubation.

In the first RCT about the use of NIV in weaning, Nava et al. [24] randomized 50 COPD patients—after a failed spontaneous breathing test—to continue intubation or to NIV. The NIV group had a significant reduction of mechanical ventilation time with a shorter ICU stay, increased weaning success, and better 60-day survival without even a single case of pneumonia (compared to 25% of the intubated patients).

Girault et al. [25] planned a similar RCT with patients who failed a spontaneous breath test. The NIV group received pressure support or volume assist ventilation resulting in a 3-day reduction in intubation time. The relevant impact of NIV on weaning is stressed by Ferrer et al. [26] that used it in patients who failed 3 times a spontaneous breathing test, decreasing the mechanical ventilation and the ICU stay in addition to reducing mortality.

Vaschetto et al. [27] tested NIV in a very specific sample of patients with hypoxemic non-hypercapnic acute respiratory failure. The inclusion criterion was not the failure of extubation trial, but the ventilator settings: when intubated patient had pressure support <25 cm H_2O, PEEP 8–13 cm H_2O, and P/F 200–300 (with a FiO2 0.6), he was given NIV for weaning. This setting reduced only the invasive ventilation time, without other results.

In a Cochrane systematic review, Burns et al. [28] analysed 16 RCTs for a total of 994 participants (with a high percentage of COPD patients). NIV was compared with other modalities of weaning: the spontaneous breathing test and the progressive reduction of invasive ventilator support. Mortality was reduced in patients who underwent NIV; also ICU and hospital stay, rate of ventilator-associated pneumonia, and time of invasive ventilation were reduced. One of the limitations of this work is that a significant portion of patients (227 patients) underwent NIV weaning without having a weaning failure.

Another indisputable advantage of NIV in weaning is patient's comfort. Often, during the spontaneous breathing test, patients report severe anxiety, which can make this weaning procedure ineffective. In some cases, it is necessary to use sedative regimens, but the use of sedation in the weaning phase is associated with its failure and should not be encouraged [29]. Furthermore, many patients, despite being physiologically "ready" for extubation, are also not at ease due to intolerance to the presence of the tube.

Before starting a weaning with the support of non-invasive ventilation, it is, however, necessary that our patient meets certain requirements:

- Adequate mental status
- Spontaneous breathing
- Adequate cough
- No need for continuous tracheal aspiration
- Airway patency
- Haemodynamically stable

Although the benefits of NIV for weaning outweighed those of invasive ventilation in most studies, one of the most important findings is the obvious non-inferiority of this technique to invasive ventilation. Being able to provide effective ventilatory support without the side effects of intubation is a big plus. Once again, to obtain positive results of NIV, patients must be carefully selected because the indiscriminate use does not involve particular advantages (apart from the already mentioned one of the removal of the endotracheal tube). COPD patients appear to be the ones who benefit most from this type of weaning. Therefore, the use of NIV is recommended for weaning support in hypercapnic patients, while it does not give any significant advantage in the hypoxic patient.

14.6 Niv and High-Flow Nasal Oxygen

Maggiore et al. [30] and Hernandez et al. [31] reported that high-flow nasal oxygen is an oxygenation option that eventually may reduce the risk of re-intubation if compared with standard oxygen with two RCTs with, respectively, 105 and 527 low risk of extubation failure patients. Beside the improved oxygenation and secretions fluidification, high flow oxygen seems to increase end-expiratory lung volume, balancing intrinsic PEEP and reducing the work of breathe.

Hernandez et al. [32] planned a RCT to test high-flow oxygen vs NIV in re-intubation and post-extubation respiratory failure in high-risk patients. The 604 patients fulfilled at least one of the following conditions:

- Age > 65 yr
- Cardiac failure as the primary cause for mechanical ventilation
- Moderate to severe COPD
- APACHE II > 12 on the day of extubation
- BMI > 30
- Airway patency not guaranteed
- Inadequate cough reflex or need for frequent suctioning
- Failure at the first attempt at weaning
- Two or more comorbidities
- Long-term mechanical ventilation >7 days

Patients in the high-flow group received nasal high-flow oxygen immediately after extubation at 10 L/min, increased according to patients tolerance. FIO2 was titrated to get SpO2 > 92%. After 24 h, high-flow was stopped. Patients in NIV group were ventilated in pressure support, with both PEEP and pressure support set to get a respiratory rate of 25/min and adequate gas exchange with SpO2 > 92% and pH < 7.35. In this study the high-flow nasal oxygen was non-inferior to NIV in preventing re-intubation in patients at high risk.

Thille et al. [33] used high-flow nasal oxygen altered with NIV, compared with high-flow nasal oxygen alone, to reduce the rate of re-intubation in high-risk patients (older than 65 years or any underlying chronic cardiac or lung disease). Patients in the NIV group underwent 12 h/day of pressure support ventilation and the remaining time received high-flow oxygen. In the high-flow oxygen + NIV group, the rate of re-intubation within the first 7 days after extubation was reduced.

Nonetheless, even if high-flow nasal oxygen could be an effective alternative to standard oxygen in standard ICU patients, the preventive use of NIV remains the first-line strategy of oxygenation in patients with high risk of extubation failure.

14.7 Conclusions

The use of NIV is rapidly increasing in every settings of intensive care medicine. To date though, the main use to avoid extubation failure is to facilitate weaning, especially in COPD patient failing a spontaneous breathing test. In these patients, NIV reduces the duration of intubation, the length of stay, the pneumonia incidence, and the tracheostomy and improves patients' survival. Another relevant field of application is the preventive use in patient candidates for elective extubation, but with risk factors for extubation failure (especially in COPD). Applied immediately after extubation, NIV decreases post-extubation respiratory distress, avoids re-intubation, and improves survival. Despite these premises, NIV, on the other hand, remains irrelevant if applied as a therapy, and not as a prophylaxis, in post-extubation respiratory failure; the only patients that could have benefits are the COPD ones.

References

1. Coplin WM, Pierson DJ, Cooley KD, Newell DW, Rubenfeld GD. Implications of extubation delay in brain-injured patients meeting standard weaning criteria. Am J Respir Crit Care Med. 2000;161(5):1530–6.
2. William OMD. The Ventilator Book. First Draught Press; 2012. ISBN 10: 098529650X
3. Dang D, Johantgen ME, Pronovost PJ, Jenckes MW, Bass EB. Postoperative complications: does intensive care unit staff nursing make a difference? Heart Lung. 2002;31:219–28.
4. Amaravadi RK, Dimick JB, Pronovost PJ, Lipsett PA. ICU nurse-to-patient ratio is associated with complications and resource use after esophagectomy. Intensive Care Med. 2000;26(12):1857–62.
5. Pronovost P, Angus DC. Economics of end-of-life care in the intensive care unit. Crit Care Med. 2001;29(2):N46–51.
6. Thille AW, Boissier F, Ben-Ghezala H, et al. Easily identified at-risk patients for extubation failure may benefit from noninvasive ventilation: a prospective before-after study. Crit Care. 2016;20:48. Published 2016 Feb 26
7. de Lassence A, Alberti C, Azoulay E, Le Miere E, Cheval C, Vincent F, Cohen Y, Garrouste-Orgeas M, Adrie C, Troche G, Timsit JF, OUTCOMEREA Study Group. Impact of unplanned extubation and reintubation after weaning on nosocomial pneumonia risk

in the intensive care unit: a prospective multicenter study. Anesthesiology. 2002;97(1):148–56.

8. McCool FD, Oyieng'o DO, Koo P. The utility of diaphragm ultrasound in reducing time to extubation. Lung. 2020;198(3):499–505.

9. Ferré A, Guillot M, Lichtenstein D, Mezière G, Richard C, Teboul JL, Monnet X. Lung ultrasound allows the diagnosis of weaning-induced pulmonary oedema. Intensive Care Med. 2019;45(5):601–8.

10. Bach JR, Saporito LR. Criteria for extubation and tracheostomy tube removal for patients with ventilatory failure. A different approach to weaning. Chest. 1996;110(6):1566–71.

11. Duan J, Han X, Huang S, Bai L. Noninvasive ventilation for avoidance of reintubation in patients with various cough strength. Crit Care. 2016;20(1):316.

12. Jiang JS, Kao SJ, Wang SN. Effect of early application of biphasic positive airway pressure on the outcome of extubation in ventilator weaning. Respirology. 1999;4(2):161–5.

13. Su CL, Chiang LL, Yang SH, Lin HI, Cheng KC, Huang YC, Wu CP. Preventive use of noninvasive ventilation after extubation: a prospective, multicenter randomized controlled trial. Respir Care. 2012;57(2):204–10.

14. Nava S, Gregoretti C, Fanfulla F, Squadrone E, Grassi M, Carlucci A, Beltrame F, Navalesi P. Noninvasive ventilation to prevent respiratory failure after extubation in high-risk patients. Crit Care Med. 2005;33(11):2465–70.

15. Ferrer M, Valencia M, Nicolas JM, Bernadich O, Badia JR, Torres A. Early noninvasive ventilation averts extubation failure in patients at risk: a randomized trial. Am J Respir Crit Care Med. 2006;173(2):164–70.

16. Ferrer M, Sellarés J, Valencia M, Carrillo A, Gonzalez G, Badia JR, Nicolas JM, Torres A. Non-invasive ventilation after extubation in hypercapnic patients with chronic respiratory disorders: randomised controlled trial. Lancet. 2009;374(9695):1082–8.

17. El-Solh AA, Aquilina A, Pineda L, Dhanvantri V, Grant B, Bouquin P. Noninvasive ventilation for prevention of post-extubation respiratory failure in obese patients. Eur Respir J. 2006;28(3):588–95. https://doi.org/10.1183/09031936.06.00150705. Epub 2006 May 31

18. Keenan SP, Powers C, McCormack DG, Block G. Noninvasive positive-pressure ventilation for postextubation respiratory distress: a randomized controlled trial. JAMA. 2002;287(24):3238–44.

19. Esteban A, Frutos-Vivar F, Ferguson ND, Arabi Y, Apezteguía C, González M, Epstein SK, Hill NS, Nava S, Soares MA, D'Empaire G, Alía I, Anzueto A. Noninvasive positive-pressure ventilation for respiratory failure after extubation. N Engl J Med. 2004;350(24):2452–60.

20. Lin C, Yu H, Fan H, Li Z. The efficacy of noninvasive ventilation in managing postextubation respiratory failure: a meta-analysis. Heart Lung. 2014;43(2):99–104.

21. Girault C, Bubenheim M, Abroug F, Diehl JL, Elatrous S, Beuret P, Richecoeur J, l'Her E, Hilbert G, Capellier G, Rabbat A, Besbes M, Guérin C, Guiot P, Bénichou J, Bonmarchand G, VENISE Trial Group. Noninvasive ventilation and weaning in patients with chronic hypercapnic respiratory failure: a randomized multicenter trial. Am J Respir Crit Care Med. 2011;184(6):672–9.

22. Kilger E, Briegel J, Haller M, Frey L, Schelling G, Stoll C, Pichler B, Peter K. Effects of noninvasive positive pressure ventilatory support in non-COPD patients with acute respiratory insufficiency after early extubation. Intensive Care Med. 1999;25(12):1374–80.

23. Vitacca M, Vianello A, Colombo D, Clini E, Porta R, Bianchi L, Arcaro G, Vitale G, Guffanti E, Lo Coco A, Ambrosino N. Comparison of two methods for weaning patients with chronic obstructive pulmonary disease requiring mechanical ventilation for more than 15 days. Am J Respir Crit Care Med. 2001;164(2):225–30.

24. Nava S, Ambrosino N, Clini E, Prato M, Orlando G, Vitacca M, Brigada P, Fracchia C, Rubini F. Noninvasive mechanical ventilation in the weaning of patients with respiratory failure due to chronic obstructive pulmonary disease. A randomized, controlled trial. Ann Intern Med. 1998;128(9):721–8.

25. Girault C, Daudenthun I, Chevron V, Tamion F, Leroy J, Bonmarchand G. Noninvasive ventilation as a systematic extubation and weaning technique in acute-on-chronic respiratory failure: a prospective, randomized controlled study. Am J Respir Crit Care Med. 1999;160(1):86–92.

26. Ferrer M, Esquinas A, Leon M, Gonzalez G, Alarcon A, Torres A. Noninvasive ventilation in severe hypoxemic respiratory failure: a randomized clinical trial. Am J Respir Crit Care Med. 2003;168(12):1438–44.

27. Vaschetto R, Turucz E, Dellapiazza F, Guido S, Colombo D, Cammarota G, Della Corte F, Antonelli M, Navalesi P. Noninvasive ventilation after early extubation in patients recovering from hypoxemic acute respiratory failure: a single-Centre feasibility study. Intensive Care Med. 2012;38(10):1599–606.

28. Burns KE, Meade MO, Premji A, Adhikari NK. Noninvasive ventilation as a weaning strategy for mechanical ventilation in adults with respiratory failure: a Cochrane systematic review. CMAJ. 2014;186(3):E112–22.

29. Conti G, Mantz J, Longrois D, Tonner P. Sedation and weaning from mechanical ventilation: time for 'best practice' to catch up with new realities? Multidiscip Respir Med. 2014;9(1):45. Published 2014 Aug 29

30. Maggiore SM, Idone FA, Vaschetto R, Festa R, Cataldo A, Antonicelli F, Montini L, De Gaetano A, Navalesi P, Antonelli M. Nasal high-flow versus venturi mask oxygen therapy after extubation. Effects on oxygenation, comfort, and clinical outcome. Am J Respir Crit Care Med. 2014;190(3):282–8.

31. Hernández G, Vaquero C, González P, Subira C, Frutos-Vivar F, Rialp G, Laborda C, Colinas L, Cuena R, Fernández R. Effect of postextubation high-flow

nasal cannula vs conventional oxygen therapy on reintubation in low-risk patients: a randomized clinical trial. JAMA. 2016;315(13):1354–61.

32. Hernández G, Vaquero C, Colinas L, et al. Effect of postextubation high-flow nasal cannula vs noninvasive ventilation on reintubation and postextubation respiratory failure in high-risk patients: a randomized clinical trial. JAMA. 2016;316(15):1565–74.

33. Thille AW, Muller G, Gacouin A, Coudroy R, Decavèle M, Sonneville R, Beloncle F, Girault C, Dangers L, Lautrette A, Cabasson S, Rouzé A, Vivier E, Le Meur A, Ricard JD, Razazi K, Barberet G, Lebert C, Ehrmann S, Sabatier C, Bourenne J, Pradel G, Bailly P, Terzi N, Dellamonica J, Lacave G, Danin PÉ, Nanadoumgar H, Gibelin A, Zanre L, Deye N, Demoule A, Maamar A, Nay MA, Robert R, Ragot S, Frat JP, HIGH-WEAN Study Group and the REVA Research Network. Effect of postextubation high-flow nasal oxygen with noninvasive ventilation vs high-flow nasal oxygen alone on reintubation among patients at high risk of extubation failure: a randomized clinical trial. JAMA. 2019;322(15):1465–75.

Critical Care Applications of NIMV and Related Issues: Intra- and Postoperative Indications for Non-invasive Mechanical Ventilation

Use of Non-invasive Ventilation in Postoperative Patients in Cardiac and Thoracic Surgeries

Marco Rispoli and Maurizio Ferrara

Contents

15.1 Postoperative Pulmonary Complications in Cardiac and Thoracic Surgeries

Cardiothoracic and thoracic surgery postoperative pulmonary complications (PPCs) are common. The need for a rapid and effective therapeutic intervention is motivated by the rapid evolution towards acute respiratory failure (ARF) in case of non-diagnosis, just like the hidden part of an iceberg: clinicians notice it when the ARF emerges, but the most dangerous part often remains hidden until too late. PPCs have a relevant impact on the postoperative course and may require re-intubation, ICU stay or mechanical ventilation causing worst outcomes, longer overall hospital stay, and lower survival.

Unfortunately, it is difficult to establish the exact incidence of PPCs, due to the unequivocal definition according to the medical literature, which varies from 2% to 40% [1, 2]. Patients undergoing cardiothoracic surgery or thoracotomy for lung resection are more prone to PPCs ranging from 8% for the first ones and 16% for the second ones.

Certain physiological conditions, previous pathological states, and the type of anesthesia and surgery may represent risk factors for the development of PPCs [3].

Patient factors
- Smoking
- 60 years old
- COPD or restrictive disease
- Cardiovascular disease
- OSAS

M. Rispoli (✉)
Department of Critical Care, Anesthesia and Intensive Care, AO dei Colli, Monaldi Hospital, Naples, Italy
e-mail: marco.rispoli@ospedalideicolli.it

M. Ferrara
Anesthesia and Critical Care, ASL Napoli 1 centro, San Paolo Hospital, Naples, Italy
e-mail: maurizio.ferrara@aslnapoli1centro.it

- Malnutrition (included obesity)
- ASA > II

Surgical factors
- Cardiopulmonary bypass
- Long surgery time
- Thoracotomy
- Diaphragm alteration
- Prolonged lungs manipulation

Anesthetic factors
- Severe postoperative pain
- Prolonged one lung ventilation
- Excessive depth of anesthesia
- Postoperative residual curarization
- Prolonged mechanical ventilation time

Even if there is still no consensus about the proper definition of PPCs, pleural effusion, diaphragmatic dysfunction, pneumonia, acute respiratory distress syndrome, pulmonary edema, and aspiration are the most common ones. All these pathological alterations lead to hypoventilation phenomena that culminate in atelectasis that is the pathophysiological basis on which ARF almost always develops.

In fact atelectasis is reported in 90% of patients after surgery due to compression of parenchymal lung and surfactant function impairment; if several risk factors coexist, the functional residual capacity can decrease up to 20–30% of the base line. Considering atelectasis as the underlying event of PPCs, it is not surprising that among the risk factors there is an inadequate control of postoperative pain that prevents the patient from being rapidly mobilized and reduces his participation in post-operative physiotherapy programs [4, 5]. But, similarly, an excessive opioid administration can determine low respiratory rate and hypoventilation, leading to hypercapnic respiratory failure.

With restoration of acceptable work of breathing being the primary therapeutic measure for atelectasis, it is not surprising that NIV is seen as a useful resource in the management of such patients considering its beneficial effects:

- Tidal volume improvement
- Collapsed alveoli recruitment
- Gas exchange optimization
- Respiratory muscles unload
- Cardiac pump optimization

One of the main problems regarding the NIV use in postoperative ARF is that it occurs typically 48–72 h after surgery, and therefore, almost always outside the ICU and this can prevent timely use because not all ordinary surgical departments are equipped with this resource, knowledge, and expertise.

15.2 Niv and Cardiothoracic Surgery

In the cardiothoracic surgery patients, postoperative ARF is the main cause of readmission in ICU with an incidence ranging from 5% to 20%. Although the postoperative restrictive pattern is inferior to that of abdominal or thoracotomy surgery, diaphragmatic dysfunction is strongly present decreasing FEV1 and vital capacity up to 65% in the first postoperative days [6]. Such ARF is associated with high Euro SCORE values, longer bypass times, and a history of renal failure. Underlying the hypoxia that characterizes such organ failure is commonly atelectasis or postoperative cardiac failure [1, 2]. As a matter of fact, emergency postoperative re-intubation due to ARF is needed in 8% of cases, increasing the mortality by 40% [1].

In cardiac surgery, postoperative hypoxia may be present even in absence of ARF and is more common in case of [7]:

- Preoperative hypoxemia
- Elevated BMI
- High transfusion requirements
- Prolonged circulatory arrest

In these patients, NIV has been applied prophylactically in the absence of ARF to improve oxygenation and reduce the work of breathing [5].

Prophylactic NIV should be used for patients presenting risk factors for postoperative hypoxemia or ARF aiming to prevent PPCs. Unluckily, as previously stated, preventive NIV cannot be applied in all cardiothoracic patients because NIV effectiveness depends on the selection of high-risk patients [5]. Early studies of preventive NIV in cardiothoracic surgery showed steady improvement in oxygenation, but mixed results in terms of reduction of atelectasis. No particular difference was reported by Matte et al. [8] in their comparison of NIV versus CPAP: the NIV group of patients received ventilation with support pressure of 12 cmH_2O with a PEEP of 5 cmH_2O, while the other group only PEEP. Pasquina et al. [9] found signs of radiological atelectasis improvement in patients receiving NIV compared to CPAP, but no relevant clinical outcomes were described. Zarbock et al. [10] tested 500 patients with nasal CPAP (10 cmH_2O) for at least 6 h per day versus standard postoperative oxygen therapy with up to 60 min per day of intermittent nasal CPAP. The authors reported a significant reduction in terms of oxygenation, need for re-intubation, pneumonia, and hospitalization in the ICU, pointing to this success as dependent on the higher CPAP settings compared to previous studies.

Liu et al. [11] performed a meta-analysis on prophylactic use of NIV in cardiac surgery: ten studies (1011 patients) were included and authors stated that atelectasis rate was lower in the patients receiving prophylactic-NIV (especially in patients >60 y-old, with preoperative hypoxia and treated with a pressure support) compared to patients receiving standard postoperative care. Moreover, prophylactic NIV could lower the rate of atelectasis, re-intubation, and other respiratory complications such as pleural effusion, pneumonia, and hypoxia, although the effect on cardiac and distal organ complications and hospital mortality might be limited.

The use of NIV for therapeutic purposes in ARF in the cardiac surgical patient is based on the assumption that it improves alveolar ventilation and gas exchange by increasing lung volumes and decreasing work of breathing. In addition, NIV decreases preload by reducing venous return; it also decreases left ventricular afterload by reducing transmural pressure and increases cardiac output. Coimbra et al. [12] included in a trail 57 cardiothoracic patients with at least three of the five following signs and symptoms:

- Dyspnoea
- Respiratory rate > 25 rpm
- Use of accessory muscles
- SpO2 < 95% with O2 5 L/min
- Chest X-ray abnormalities in at least two quadrants

The postoperative NIV avoided re-intubation in 54% of the cases. Although patients received three different NIV modalities, no statistically significant difference among them was reported, but a better trend with the use of two-pressure level modalities. In the CPAP modality, there was a greater number of re-intubations, even though the difference between the groups was not significant. Anyway, the scientific literature reported no consistent data about efficacy and safety of NIV in postoperative cardiothoracic patients. In a recent meta-analyses, Zhu et al. [13] reported data from 14 RCTs (1740 patients), providing evidence supporting the protective role of NIV in specific patient subpopulations: "Overall, NIV played an important role in determining patients' need for endotracheal intubation and respiratory complications, respiratory rate, and pH in patients undergoing cardiac surgery. Furthermore, NIV showed a significant effect on mortality, respiratory and heart rate, PaO_2/FiO_2 ratio, and pH in patients undergoing pulmonary surgery. No other significant effect was observed based on disease status".

Ampatzidou et al. [14] retrospectively identified the presence of COPD, low preoperative renal function, higher BMI, and high Euro-SCORE II as independent characteristics of patient subpopulations needing NIV for postoperative ARF.

The use of NIV should be encouraged even in ordinary surgical ward outside ICU, as Olper et al. [15] reported a successful 3-day CPAP cycle of treatment in cardiac surgery ward with improved respiratory outcome. This aspect is often overlooked in the application of NIV, but while ARF is more likely to develop outside the ICU due to timing greater than 48 h, on the other hand late application of NIV can delay the possible re-intubation with increased mortality.

Lately, the use of high-flow oxygen therapy has spread to ICUs, proving to guarantee good results when used as prophylaxis in patients with low and high risk of re-intubation [16]. Some authors report non-inferiority results with respect to NIV, while others used intermittent cycles of high-flow oxygen and NIV [17]. Zochios et al. [18] tested in a RCT the impact of high nasal flow oxygen (HFNC) on 100 cardiac surgery candidate patients at high risk of re-intubation. They compared the use of HFNC versus traditional oxygen therapy immediately after extubation for 24 h. Patients recruited had COPD, asthma, recent lower respiratory tract infection, strong smoking addiction, or morbidly obesity. Authors reported a significant reduction in hospital stay.

However, a recent meta-analysis conducted by Lu et al. [19] on 1327 patients reported a significantly lower re-intubation rate and rate of escalation of respiratory support compared with standard oxygen therapy in post-extubation adult surgical patients, but there is no difference in the incidence of PPCs or mortality. Lu et al. subgroup analyses showed no improvement in the re-intubation rate in patients who had undergone cardiac surgery and received HFNC compared with standard oxygen therapy post-extubation.

15.3 NIV and Thoracic Surgery

Regarding what concerns thoracic surgery, the pathophysiological timing of atelectasis development is common to that of cardiac surgery. The main difference lies in the typical characteristics of the lung cancer patients who commonly suffer from COPD, so the possibility of weaning may be more difficult. On the other hand, recent lung resection, if subjected to NIV, may result in the development or worsening of air leakage, and therefore this factor must be added to the decision-making balance.

An important and recent experience on the use of prophylactic NIV in thoracic surgery comes from Paleiron et al. [26] who selected 300 patients undergoing lung resective surgery considered at high-risk of PPCs: obstructive or restrictive lung disease, recent hypercapnic ARF, oxygen therapy, heart failure, history of acute cardiogenic edema, or obesity. One hundred fifty-three patients started NIV 6 h/day from 15 days to 7 days before thoracic surgery. In this study, preoperative NIV did not decrease the postoperative complication rate after lung cancer surgery nor multivariable analysis adjusted on type of surgery, COPD, and diffusion alteration did change this result.

The Italian intersociety consensus on Perioperative Anaesthesia Care in Thoracic surgery [22] does not recommend the NIV routine use to prevent PPCS, prolonged length of stay, and mortality in patients undergoing major thoracic surgery. This approach could be considered on a case by case basis in selected high-risk patients (obese patients or patients with COPD, obese, chronic heart failure, or chronic hypersecretion) [23, 24].

Auriant et al. [20] enrolled 24 patients who underwent lung respective surgery with at least three of the following: respiratory rate $\geq$ 25 bpm, use of accessory respiratory muscles, PaO_2/FiO_2 ratio < 200, or chest radiography abnormalities. Patients were randomly assigned to standard oxygen treatment or with NIV to achieve a tidal volume of 8–10 mL/kg with a respiratory rate <25 bpm: patients treated with NIV had reduction in need for re-intubation, in-hospital, and 3-month mortality. Torres et al. [21] performed a meta-analysis on a total of 486 patients, reporting that no additional benefit was provided by NIV in terms of PPCs reduction, rate of intubation, mortality, postoperative consumption of antibiotics, length of ICU stay, length of hospital stay, and adverse effects related to NIV. Such an approach should be carefully weighed as it has been documented by Riviere et al. [25] that NIV failure, occurring in approximately 20% of patients, is related with increase in terms of pneumonia and mortality. According to Riviere et al. the independent NIV failure risk factors are: increase of respiratory rate, SOFA score increase, number of fiberoptic bronchoscopies, and number of hours in NIV.

For this reason, it may be useful to stratify the "high-risk of NIV failure patients" in order to identify those who may benefit from NIV and those who should be referred directly to re-intubation. Anyway, the Italian intersociety consensus on Perioperative Anaesthesia Care in Thoracic surgery [22] recommends the use of NIV or CPAP to treat acute respiratory failure complicating thoracic surgery; furthermore, the use of HFNC as an alternative or integrative support to CPAP or NIV is still viable to treat ARF in thoracic surgery.

15.4   Conclusion

The lack of evidence in NIV protocols and the differences in patient comorbidities make particularly difficult to identify strong evidence regarding the prophylactic or therapeutic use of NIV in patients who are candidates for cardiac and thoracic surgery. Probably, just as with any other area of NIV application, the benefits are relevant only to specific categories of patients, and indiscriminate use does not allow the different nuances to be captured. In addition, a delay in the eventual re-intubation of patients who have undergone major surgeries, such as cardiothoracic surgeries, may translate into a significant increase in mortality if we overly dwell on non-invasive ventilatory support. Actually, the use of NIV to treat postoperative ARF is recommended, while the prophylactic use must be reserved to selected patients.

References

1. Cabrini L, Zangrillo A, Landoni G. Preventive and therapeutic non-invasive ventilation in cardiovascular surgery. Curr Opin Anaesthesiol. 2015;28:67–72.
2. Gilliland S, Brainard J. Postoperative non-invasive ventilation following cardiothoracic surgery: a clinical primer and review of the literature. Semin Cardiothorac Vasc Anesth. 2015;19:302–8.
3. Esquinas AM, Jover JL, Úbeda A, et al. Non-invasive mechanical ventilation in the pre- and intraoperative period and difficult airway. Rev Esp Anestesiol Reanim. 2015;62:502–11.
4. Pieczkoski SM, Margarites AGF, Sbruzzi G. Non-invasive ventilation during immediate postoperative period in cardiac surgery patients: systematic review and meta-analysis. Braz J Cardiovasc Surg. 2017;32:301–11.
5. Al Jaaly E, Fiorentino F, Reeves BC, et al. Effect of adding postoperative non-invasive ventilation to usual care to prevent pulmonary complications in patients undergoing coronary artery bypass grafting: a randomised controlled trial. J Thorac Cardiovasc Surg. 2013;146:912–8.
6. Warner DO, Weiskopf RB. Preventing postoperative pulmonary complications: the role of the anesthesiologist. Anesthesiology. 2000;92:1467–72.
7. Yang Y, Sun L, Liu N, et al. Effects of non-invasive positive-pressure ventilation with different interfaces in patients with hypoxemia after surgery for Stanford type a aortic dissection. Med Sci Monit. 2015;21:2294–304.
8. Matte P, Jacquet L, Van Dyck M, Goenen M. Effects of conventional physiotherapy, continuous positive airway pressure and non-invasive ventilatory support with bilevel positive airway pressure after coronary artery bypass grafting. Acta Anaesthesiol Scand. 2000;44(1):75–81.
9. Pasquina P, Merlani P, Granier JM, Ricou B. Continuous positive airway pressure versus noninvasive pressure support ventilation to treat atelectasis after cardiac surgery. Anesth Analg. 2004;99(4):1001–8.
10. Zarbock A, Mueller E, Netzer S, Gabriel A, Feindt P, Kindgen-Milles D. Prophylactic nasal continuous positive airway pressure following cardiac surgery protects from postoperative pulmonary complications: a prospective, randomized, controlled trial in 500 patients. Chest. 2009;135(5):1252–9.
11. Liu Q, Shan M, Liu J, Cui L, Lan C. Prophylactic noninvasive ventilation versus conventional care in patients after cardiac surgery. J Surg Res. 2020;246:384–94.
12. Coimbra VR, Lara Rde A, Flores EG, Nozawa E, Auler JO Jr, Feltrim MI. Application of noninvasive ventilation in acute respiratory failure after cardiovascular surgery. Arq Bras Cardiol. 2007;89(5):270–6. 298–305
13. Zhu G, Huang Y, Wei D, Shi Y. Efficacy and safety of noninvasive ventilation in patients after cardiothoracic surgery: a PRISMA-compliant systematic review and meta-analysis. Medicine (Baltimore). 2016;95(38):e4734.
14. Ampatzidou F, Boutou AK, Karagounis L, Marczin N, Gogakos A, Drossos G. Noninvasive ventilation to treat respiratory failure after cardiac surgery: predictors of application and outcome. Respir Care. 2019;64(9):1123–31.

15. Olper L, Bignami E, Di Prima AL, Albini S, Nascimbene S, Cabrini L, Landoni G, Alfieri O. Continuous positive airway pressure versus oxygen therapy in the cardiac surgical ward: a randomized trial. J Cardiothorac Vasc Anesth. 2017;31(1):115–21.

16. Hernández G, Vaquero C, Colinas L, et al. Effect of postextubation high-flow nasal cannula vs noninvasive ventilation on reintubation and postextubation respiratory failure in high-risk patients: a randomized clinical trial. JAMA. 2016;316(15):1565–74.

17. Thille AW, Muller G, Gacouin A, Coudroy R, Decavèle M, Sonneville R, Beloncle F, Girault C, Dangers L, Lautrette A, Cabasson S, Rouzé A, Vivier E, Le Meur A, Ricard JD, Razazi K, Barberet G, Lebert C, Ehrmann S, Sabatier C, Bourenne J, Pradel G, Bailly P, Terzi N, Dellamonica J, Lacave G, Danin PÉ, Nanadoumgar H, Gibelin A, Zanre L, Deye N, Demoule A, Maamar A, Nay MA, Robert R, Ragot S, Frat JP, HIGH-WEAN Study Group and the REVA Research Network. Effect of postextubation high-flow nasal oxygen with noninvasive ventilation vs high-flow nasal oxygen alone on reintubation among patients at high risk of extubation failure: a randomized clinical trial. JAMA. 2019;322(15):1465–75.

18. Zochios V, Collier T, Blaudszun G, Butchart A, Earwaker M, Jones N, Klein AA. The effect of high-flow nasal oxygen on hospital length of stay in cardiac surgical patients at high risk for respiratory complications: a randomised controlled trial. Anaesthesia. 2018;73(12):1478–88.

19. Lu Z, Chang W, Meng SS, Zhang X, Xie J, Xu JY, Qiu H, Yang Y, Guo F. Effect of high-flow nasal cannula oxygen therapy compared with conventional oxygen therapy in postoperative patients: a systematic review and meta-analysis. BMJ Open. 2019;9(8):e027523.

20. Auriant I, Jallot A, Hervé P, Cerrina J, Le Roy LF, Fournier JL, Lescot B, Parquin F. Noninvasive ventilation reduces mortality in acute respiratory failure following lung resection. Am J Respir Crit Care Med. 2001;164(7):1231–5.

21. Torres MF, Porfírio GJ, Carvalho AP, Riera R. Noninvasive positive pressure ventilation for prevention of complications after pulmonary resection in lung cancer patients. Cochrane Database Syst Rev. 2019;3(3):CD010355.

22. Piccioni F, Droghetti A, Bertani A, et al. Recommendations from the Italian intersociety consensus on perioperative anesthesa care in thoracic surgery (PACTS) part 2: intraoperative and postoperative care. Perioper Med (Lond). 2020;9:31. Published 2020 Oct 23

23. Rochwerg B, Brochard L, Elliott MW, Hess D, Hill NS, Nava S, et al. Official ERS/ATS clinical practice guidelines: noninvasive ventilation for acute respiratory failure. Eur Respir J. 2017;50(2):1602426.

24. Scala R, Pisani L. Noninvasive ventilation in acute respiratory failure: which recipe for success? Eur Respir Rev. 2018;27(149):180029.

25. Riviere S, Monconduit J, Zarka V, Massabie P, Boulet S, Dartevelle P, et al. Failure of noninvasive ventilation after lung surgery: a comprehensive analysis of incidence and possible risk factors. Eur J Cardiothorac Surg. 2011;39:769–76.

26. Paleiron N, Grassin F, Lancelin C, Tromeur C, Margery J, Natale C, Couturaud F, GFPC Group. Assessment of preoperative noninvasive ventilation before lung cancer surgery: the preOVNI randomized controlled study. J Thorac Cardiovasc Surg. 2020;160(4):1050–1059.e3.

Use of Non-invasive Ventilation in Postoperative Patients in Abdominal Surgery

Yuda Sutherasan, Akarawut Kasemchaiyanun, and Pongdhep Theerawit

Contents

Y. Sutherasan (✉)
Division of Pulmonary and Pulmonary Critical Care
Medicine, Department of Medicine Ramathibodi
Hospital, Faculty of Medicine Ramathibodi Hospital,
Mahidol University, Bangkok, Thailand

A. Kasemchaiyanun · P. Theerawit
Division of Critical Care Medicine, Department of
Medicine Ramathibodi Hospital, Faculty of Medicine
Ramathibodi Hospital, Mahidol University,
Bangkok, Thailand

16.1   Introduction

Postoperative pulmonary complications (PPCs) are defined as pulmonary abnormalities occurring in the postoperative period. It has been reported that 3.4–40% of patients undergoing abdominal surgery developed at least one of PPCs [1, 2]. PPCs *include the following conditions*: (1) postoperative pneumonia; (2) pulmonary edema; (3) atelectasis; (4) hypoxemia; (5) bronchospasm; (6) fever; (7) acute respiratory distress syndrome (ARDS); and (8) acute respiratory failure (ARF). Those complications may

© The Author(s), under exclusive license to Springer Nature Switzerland AG 2023
G. Servillo, M. Vargas (eds.), *Non-invasive Mechanical Ventilation in Critical Care, Anesthesiology and Palliative Care*, https://doi.org/10.1007/978-3-031-36510-2_16

increase the need for invasive mechanical ventilation, length of hospital stay (LOS), and mortality [2]. Non-invasive ventilation (NIV) is the respiratory support that could prevent endotracheal intubations and invasive ventilation complications.

Our chapter aims to describe the mechanisms, risk factors of PPCs, the rationales, benefits, and practical aspects of NIV application during the perioperative period in abdominal surgery to prevent or treat PPCs.

16.2 Risk Factors and Mechanisms of Abdominal Surgery-Induced Postoperative Pulmonary Complications

The risk factors associated with PPCs were operative procedure, general anesthesia, the incision-site, the duration of anesthesia of more than 3.5 h, and host factors such as older age, American Society of Anesthesiologists (ASA) functional status II or greater, chronic obstructive pulmonary disease, obstructive sleep apnea (OSA), cardiovascular disease, impaired preoperative cognitive function, smoking history within the past 8 weeks, overweight, and history of cancer [3].

There are several mechanisms related to PPCs in post-abdominal surgery. General anesthesia (GA) reduces respiratory drive of the muscular tone, impairs the cough ability, and the physiologic response to hypoxia and hypercapnia. Upper abdominal and thoracic surgery is associated with the reduction of lung volume. The trauma during abdominal surgery near the diaphragm disturbs the abdominal muscle and thoracic wall and the forces of the diaphragm. The procedure aggravates the pain, diminishes the activity of phrenic and respiratory muscle nerves [4], and disrupts regular coordination of respiratory muscle function, leading to a decrease in functional residual capacity (FRC) and vital capacity for several days after surgery. The reduction of FRC by compression of lung tissue impairs surfactant function, causing atelectasis in

dependent lung regions [5]. The prolonged period with a high concentration of oxygen during GA may produce absorptive atelectasis.

Furthermore, the occurrence of atelectasis is risky to pneumonia [3]. These intraoperative disturbances of the breathing mechanisms can persist in the postoperative period [5]. Postoperative ARDS could occur and shared similar pathophysiology as ARDS. Pro-inflammatory cytokines and cytokines, i.e., interleukin (IL) 1 beta, IL-6, and IL 8, and damage-associated molecular patterns of molecules, have been shown to play roles in postoperative acute lung injury [6].

Applying NIV could yield benefits in PPCs, namely, increase in FRC and reduction of ventilation-perfusion mismatch, atelectasis and work of breathing, and avoiding the need for endotracheal intubation [2].

16.3 Role of Non-invasive Ventilation in Abdominal Surgery

16.3.1 Prevention of Postoperative Pulmonary Complications

Recently, NIV in the postoperative setting has been established in a guideline [7]. However, the recent guideline has recommended using the NIV, either continuous positive airway pressure (CPAP) or Bi-level positive airway pressure (BiPAP), in postoperative patients with ARF.

Carlsson et al. had given 4-h CPAP (5–10 cm H_2O) via facemask to patients undergoing post-cholecystectomy. The primary outcomes showed no significant difference regarding PPCs [8]. However, an randomized controlled trial (RCT) by Joris et al. in 1997 conducted in obese patients undergoing abdominal surgery demonstrated the significant improvement of Force vital capacity (FVC), Forced expiratory volume in 1 s (FEV1), and SpO_2 in the group receiving BiPAP. In 2002, Ebeo et al. researched the benefit of NIV regarding physiologic and clinical outcomes. This study randomized patients to receiving the NIV or oxygen therapy [9]. Despite a significant improvement of FVC, FEV1, and SpO_2 in the NIV group, the differences in LOS or PPCs were not demonstrated.

A study in Brazil by Baltieri et al. revealed a prevalence of atelectasis as high as 37% in patients undergoing bariatric surgery [10]. Ricksten et al. studied an RCT in elective upper abdominal surgery [11]. They compared CPAP, positive expiratory pressure (PEP), and deep-breathing device postoperatively. Their results showed a lower rate of atelectasis in CPAP and PEP than in the deep-breathing device group. An RCT by Rocha et al. compared the effect of BiPAP versus inspiratory load exercise after bariatric surgery [12]. The BiPAP was set to IPAP by 12 cm H_2O and EPAP by 8 cm H_2O, immediately at the recovery room and intermittently afterward. There was no significant difference regarding the presence of atelectasis between groups.

The role of NIV in preventing postoperative pneumonia was demonstrated [13]. A study by Denehy et al. showed a lower proportion of patients developing new pulmonary opacity in the postoperative NIV group but not reached statistical significance [14]. A significantly lower rate of pneumonia was reported in Squadrone et al. [15] study, showing 2% of patients with pneumonia in the NIV group and 10% in the group using oxygen therapy. Also, the benefit of NIV regarding ICU-acquired pneumonia (IAP) was reported in a recent RCT. The rate of IAP in the NIV group was 14.6%, significantly lower than 29.7% in standard oxygen therapy [16].

The prophylaxis NIV for reintubation is rational after abdominal surgery. Olsen et al. conducted an RCT in 70 patients undergoing thoracoabdominal surgery. The patients were randomly assigned to CPAP or inspiratory resistance-positive expiratory pressure (IR-PEP) [17]. The CPAP level ranged from 5 cm to 10 cm H_2O and lasted 30 min every 2 h during the first 3 days after the operation. The reintubation was significantly lower in patients assigned to CPAP therapy than in the IR-PEP. This result is consistent with another RCT by Squadrone et al. This study enrolled patients undergoing major elective abdominal surgery developing severe hypoxemia [15]. They compared oxygen therapy via venturi mask, FiO_2 0.5 versus oxygen FiO_2 0.5 plus CPAP 7.5 cm H_2O. A substantially lower intubation rate was observed in the CPAP group than in the oxygen therapy group.

Regarding overall PPCs, the comparison between CPAP versus physiotherapy has been made. Denehy et al. conducted an RCT studying the effect of physiotherapy compared with CPAP by 10 cm H_2O plus physiotherapy in various abdominal surgeries [14]. The percentage of PPCs in the CPAP group was lower than the control group, but the statistical analysis could not be determined due to the low prevalence of overall PPCs. Lockstone et al. conducted a pre-post study in high-risk elective upper abdominal surgery, comparing prevalence of PPCs in a cohort-prescribed 2-day NIV with standard postoperative physiotherapy [18]. The results showed the reduction of PPC from 18% to 7% in the NIV group. In addition, an ongoing RCT by Lockstone et al. has been conducted in high-risk upper abdominal surgical patients, comparing usual care versus usual care plus five 30-min NIV session for the first 48 h after surgery [19]. The primary outcome has been the postoperative pulmonary complication during the first 14 postoperative days. Even though the results from previous trials have not confirmed the benefits of NIV regarding PPCs reduction, the postoperative NIV after abdominal surgery provides a potential role from a meta-analysis [20].

The prophylaxis NIV has a role in postoperative abdominal surgery. It prevents patients from hypoxemia, atelectasis, pulmonary infection, and reintubation. In addition, it provides a potential role for the prevention of overall PPC.

16.3.2 Treatment of Postoperative Pulmonary Complications

Postoperative hypoxemia is not uncommon. It may become severe and persistent [21]. The risk factor associated with this event is the surgical site. Since 1999, an observational study by Xue et al. has demonstrated the evolution of pulse oximetry after a 3-h postoperative period of three operations [22]. This study revealed the lowest desaturation in thoracoabdominal surgery, followed by upper abdominal surgery.

Recently, the CPAP has been shown to improve postoperative hypoxemic complications. This study randomized 209 elective abdominal surgical patients developing postoperative hypoxemia to receive the CPAP plus oxygen or oxygen therapy [15]. The primary outcome showed a lower intubation rate in the CPAP group than in the control group. Furthermore, the rate of pneumonia and sepsis also decreases compared to the control group.

Jaber et al. confirmed the benefit of CPAP in abdominal surgery having postoperative hypoxemia [16]. They included elective and non-elective cases and randomly provided the BiPAP via facemask plus oxygen therapy or oxygen therapy alone to participants. This study reported a significantly lower reintubation rate during 7-day post operation in the BiPAP group. Also, the invasive ventilation-free day and hospital-acquired infection rates were different. However, the 90-day mortality was similar.

The incidence of postoperative atelectasis is previously discussed. Physiologically, providing CPAP should correct this complication. In 2008, a meta-analysis by Ferreyra et al. included five studies to analyze the benefit of NIV for the treatment of atelectasis after abdominal surgery. The results favored using the CPAP rather than standard therapy to treat atelectasis postoperatively [23].

The NIV in abdominal surgery improves hypoxemia and atelectasis. In addition, it prevents respiratory failure and reduces the risk of postoperative pulmonary infection.

16.3.3 Complications of NIV in Abdominal Surgery

A significant concern about postoperative NIV complications in abdominal surgery is anastomosis leakage. Interestingly, an experimental study in pigs showed exciting results. Raman et al.

studied a threshold of esophageal pressure tolerable to anastomosis leakage in the pig model [24]. The author created end-to-end esophago-gastric anastomosis and applied intraluminal pressure until the leakage was detected. The threshold pressure leading to leakage was 84 cm H_2O. While applying pressure by 40 cm H_2O via the laryngeal mask airway, the maximum esophageal pressure was 16 cm H_2O, nearly five times lower than the threshold.

A study by Denehy et al. conducted an RCT in patients undergoing abdominal surgery to determine the benefit of CPAP regarding lung function and oxygenation [14]. They included 35 colorectal surgery patients in their study. The CPAP was set by 10 cm H_2O for 15 or 30 min. Interestingly, the authors did not report the complications related to applying CPAP. Also, the research using CPAP was conducted in thoracoabdominal surgery. This study provided CPAP 5–10 cm H_2O in gastro-esophageal reconstruction. Twenty-eight patients were randomly assigned to CPAP. There was no complication reported from this study [17].

Other than CPAP, the BiPAP was applied in post abdominal surgery, namely, in a study undergoing open Roux-en Y gastric bypass in obese patients [9]. The IPAP and EPAP were set by 12 cm and 4 cm H_2O, respectively. Of 14 patients receiving BiPAP, no abdominal distension was observed in this study.

An RCT included 209 patients undergoing abdominal surgery [15]. Sixty percent of patients in the CPAP group at risk of anastomosis leakage were randomly assigned to CPAP. The CPAP was created by a high flow generating device up to 140 L/min, providing CPAP by 7.5 cm H_2O. The duration of CPAP use was 6 h. The anastomosis leakage was found in one patient in the CPAP group compared to six in the control group.

Recently, the largest RCT was conducted by Jaber et al. [16]. They enrolled 393 patients undergoing abdominal surgery in their study. In addition, the NIV group contained 71 subjects undergoing esophagus or gastrointestinal operations. The NIV was delivered via facemask and set to BiPAP. The IPAP was started at 5 cm H_2O

and increased up to 15 cm H_2O. The EPAP was set initially at 5 cm H_2O and then increased up to 10 cm H_2O. The NIV was used at least 6 h within the first 24 h postoperatively. The abdominal distension was not found, and anastomosis leakage was not reported.

Utilizing the NIV is safe in postoperative abdominal surgery. The threshold pressure regarding IPAP and EPAP was 10–15 cm and 5–10 cm H_2O, respectively, for 6 h.

16.4 Definitions and Principles of the Two Main NIV Techniques

NIV works by administration of positive airway pressure without using an invasive artificial airway. The most common modes are CPAP and BiPAP. The CPAP is a single constant fixed level of positive airway pressure throughout inspiration and expiration. While BiPAP has two airway pressure levels: one delivered during the inhalation (IPAP) and a lower one during exhalation (EPAP).

The patient's spontaneous inspiratory effort triggers the ventilator, providing a variable flow of gas delivered until the preset pressure support level is reached. Once the selected pressure support level is reached, the patient can breathe until the inspiratory flow rate drops below a threshold level (40–60% of the peak flow). Then, the ventilator will cycle to the expiratory phase.

Some machines have additional timed modes where the ventilator can be terminated to the expiratory phase when preset time intervals are achieved. A backup rate is essential in patients who had remaining effects of sedative or neuromuscular blocking agents postoperatively. Both CPAP and NIV increase recruitment of collapsed lungs, maintain patency of the upper airway, and decrease work of breathing. The main difference between BiPAP and CPAP is that BiPAP offers pressure support (PS = IPAP level minus EPAP level), allow the patient to get more alveolar ventilation and dyspnea relief. NIV should be considered in patients with combined hypercarbia and hypoxemia.

16.5 How to Set NIV and Duration of Trial

Postoperative NIV can be used in two main strategies. First, prophylactic NIV was applied to prevent postoperative ARF in patients predisposed to developing hypoxemia with or without hypercarbia (i.e., elderly, morbid obesity, obstructive sleep apnea, chronic obstructive pulmonary disease, heart disease). Second, NIV is a therapeutic option in patients with postoperative respiratory failure. Current practice guidelines suggest NIV may be an alternative to conventional ventilation in patients who had a respiratory failure during the postoperative period, while prophylactic NIV is not as clear and remains to be defined [7].

Guidance regarding the optimal timing of use had not yet been established. Optimal NIV protocol delivered (duration, interfaces, settings, etc.) remains controversial, frequently relying on the clinician's experience. The proper IPAP and EPAP, especially as a prophylactic therapy, must always be personalized conditioning. The head of a patient's bed should be elevated to 30 degrees. Ventilator settings should be checked and set before connecting to the patient using the simple following initial settings:

- NIV with a backup rate (spontaneous/timed, S/T Mode).
- Inspiratory trigger of -1 to -2 L min^{-1} or -1 to -2 cm H_2O.
- IPAP level above EPAP level of 3–5 usually cm H_2O used at initiation (IPAP + EPAP should not exceed 25 cm H_2O; if the maximal pressure is more than 25 cm H_2O, the invasive mechanical ventilation may be indicated).
- Expiratory cycling of 40–60% or fixed inspiratory time of 1 s [1:2–1:3 (Chronic obstructive pulmonary disease) or 1:1(Neuromuscular disease/Obesity hypoventilation syndrome)].
- EPAP level of 3–5 cm H_2O and FiO_2 (to maintain individualized, targeted SpO_2).

The IPAP and EPAP levels should be gradually titrated in 1–2 cm H_2O incrementally until clinical dyspnea is improved or patient tolerability and good synchrony have been reached. In addition, the following parameters should be closely monitored: (1) vital signs; (2) consciousness level; (3) pulse oximetry; (4) arterial blood gases (followed by 1-, 4-, and 6-h after initiation of NIV); (5) side effect; and (6) prompt endotracheal tube intubation in case of failure NIV.

16.6 Problems Related to NIV in Postoperative Patients in Abdominal Surgery

NIV may increase insufflation of air into the stomach and may promote gastric distension and aspiration. Historically, patients following upper gastrointestinal anastomotic surgery were a contraindication to NIV due to anastomotic breakdown induced by positive pressure. However, several studies show that NIV wasn't harmful to use in patients undergoing esophageal or gastric surgery. In addition, it may attenuate postoperative hypoxemia and decreased re-intubation incidence without increasing the risk of anastomotic leakage [25–27].

Most abdominal surgery patients have inserted a nasogastric (NG) tube during the perioperative period. Unfortunately, the NG tube insertion for those requiring NIV can be associated with some problems, such as the air leakage around the facial mask, which may reduce NIV effectiveness. However, this problem may be avoided with NIV masks with a port for NG tubes, but these are not widely available. Alternatively, we suggest padding the skin below the NG tube with silicone dressing to reduce air leakage and facial pressure sore [28]. One thing, patients with post-abdominal surgery increase susceptibility to gastric overdistension during NIV and may lead to suspending treatment; the NG tube on a bag can theoretically reduce this adverse effect.

16.7 Contraindication

Contraindications to the use of NIV following abdominal surgery did not differ from the general population. However, it is essential to exclude any contraindications to the application of NIV before being used.

Absolute Contraindications
- Impaired consciousness, severe agitation, or encephalopathy.
- A cardiac or respiratory arrest or hemodynamic instability.
- Active cardiac arrhythmia or cardiac ischemia.
- Excessive respiratory secretions.
- Severe upper gastrointestinal bleeding or hemoptysis.
- Facial trauma.
- Uncontrolled vomiting.
- Upper airway obstruction (NIV may be helpful in OSA).
- Patient declines.

Relative Contraindications
- Mildly decreased level of consciousness.
- Progressive severe respiratory failure.
- Uncooperative patients who can be calmed or comforted.
- Pregnancy.

16.8 Conclusion

Postoperative abdominal surgery in high-risk patients could increase PPCs, morbidity, and mortality. NIV in the postoperative period could prevent and treat PPCs by improving hypoxemia, atelectasis, and reducing the risk of postoperative pulmonary infection. The experience of the physician, appropriate settings, and NIV application techniques are essential when physicians decide to use the NIV.

References

1. Ávila AC, Fenili R. Incidence and risk factors for postoperative pulmonary complications in patients undergoing thoracic and abdominal surgeries. Rev Col Bras Cir. 2017;44(3):284–92.
2. Chiumello D, Chevallard G, Gregoretti C. Non-invasive ventilation in postoperative patients: a systematic review. Intensive Care Med. 2011;37(6):918–29.

3. Tusman G, Bohm SH, Warner DO, Sprung J. Atelectasis and perioperative pulmonary complications in high-risk patients. Curr Opin Anaesthesiol. 2012;25(1):1–10.
4. Canet J, Mazo V. Postoperative pulmonary complications. Minerva Anestesiol. 2010;76(2):138–43.
5. Warner DO. Preventing postoperative pulmonary complications: the role of the anesthesiologist. Anesthesiology. 2000;92(5):1467–72.
6. Chen L, Zhao H, Alam A, Mi E, Eguchi S, Yao S, et al. Postoperative remote lung injury and its impact on surgical outcome. BMC Anesthesiol. 2019;19(1):30.
7. Rochwerg B, Brochard L, Elliott MW, Hess D, Hill NS, Nava S, et al. Official ERS/ATS clinical practice guidelines: non-invasive ventilation for acute respiratory failure. Eur Respir J. 2017;50(2):1602426.
8. Carlsson C, Sonden B, Thylen U. Can postoperative continuous positive airway pressure (CPAP) prevent pulmonary complications after abdominal surgery? Intensive Care Med. 1981;7(5):225–9.
9. Ebeo CT, Benotti PN, Byrd RP Jr, Elmaghraby Z, Lui J. The effect of bi-level positive airway pressure on postoperative pulmonary function following gastric surgery for obesity. Respir Med. 2002;96(9):672–6.
10. Baltieri L, Peixoto-Souza FS, Rasera-Junior I, Montebelo MI, Costa D, Pazzianotto-Forti EM. Analysis of the prevalence of atelectasis in patients undergoing bariatric surgery. Braz J Anesthesiol. 2016;66(6):577–82.
11. Ricksten SE, Bengtsson A, Soderberg C, Thorden M, Kvist H. Effects of periodic positive airway pressure by mask on postoperative pulmonary function. Chest. 1986;89(6):774–81.
12. Rocha M, Souza S, Costa CMD, Merino DFB, Montebelo MIL, Rasera-Junior I, et al. Airway positive pressure vs. exercises with inspiratory loading focused on pulmonary and respiratory muscular functions in the postoperative period of bariatric surgery. Arq Bras Cir Dig. 2018;31(2):e1363.
13. Stock MC, Downs JB, Gauer PK, Alster JM, Imrey PB. Prevention of postoperative pulmonary complications with CPAP, incentive spirometry, and conservative therapy. Chest. 1985;87(2):151–7.
14. Denehy L, Carroll S, Ntoumenopoulos G, Jenkins S. A randomized controlled trial comparing periodic mask CPAP with physiotherapy after abdominal surgery. Physiother Res Int. 2001;6(4):236–50.
15. Squadrone V, Coha M, Cerutti E, Schellino MM, Biolino P, Occella P, et al. Continuous positive airway pressure for treatment of postoperative hypoxemia: a randomized controlled trial. JAMA. 2005;293(5):589–95.
16. Jaber S, Lescot T, Futier E, Paugam-Burtz C, Seguin P, Ferrandiere M, et al. Effect of non-invasive ventilation on tracheal reintubation among patients with hypoxemic respiratory failure following abdominal surgery: a randomized clinical trial. JAMA. 2016;315(13):1345–53.
17. Fagevik Olsen M, Wennberg E, Johnsson E, Josefson K, Lonroth H, Lundell L. Randomized clinical study of the prevention of pulmonary complications after thoracoabdominal resection by two different breathing techniques. Br J Surg. 2002;89(10):1228–34.
18. Lockstone J, Parry SM, Denehy L, Robertson IK, Story D, Parkes S, et al. Physiotherapist administered, non-invasive ventilation to reduce postoperative pulmonary complications in high-risk patients following elective upper abdominal surgery; a before-and-after cohort implementation study. Physiotherapy. 2020;106:77–86.
19. Lockstone J, Boden I, Robertson IK, Story D, Denehy L, Parry SM. Non-invasive positive airway pressure therapy to reduce postoperative lung complications following upper abdominal surgery (NIPPER PLUS): protocol for a single-centre, pilot, randomised controlled trial. BMJ Open. 2019;9(1):e023139.
20. Kokotovic D, Berkfors A, Gogenur I, Ekeloef S, Burcharth J. The effect of postoperative respiratory and mobilization interventions on postoperative complications following abdominal surgery: a systematic review and meta-analysis. Eur J Trauma Emerg Surg. 2021;47(4):975–90.
21. Sun Z, Sessler DI, Dalton JE, Devereaux PJ, Shahinyan A, Naylor AJ, et al. Postoperative hypoxemia is common and persistent: a prospective blinded observational study. Anesth Analg. 2015;121(3):709–15.
22. Xue FS, Li BW, Zhang GS, Liao X, Zhang YM, Liu JH, et al. The influence of surgical sites on early postoperative hypoxemia in adults undergoing elective surgery. Anesth Analg. 1999;88(1):213–9.
23. Ferreyra GP, Baussano I, Squadrone V, Richiardi L, Marchiaro G, Del Sorbo L, et al. Continuous positive airway pressure for treatment of respiratory complications after abdominal surgery: a systematic review and meta-analysis. Ann Surg. 2008;247(4):617–26.
24. Raman V, MacGlaflin CE, Erkmen CP. Non-invasive positive pressure ventilation following esophagectomy: safety demonstrated in a pig model. Chest. 2015;147(2):356–61.
25. Huerta S, DeShields S, Shpiner R, Li Z, Liu C, Sawicki M, et al. Safety and efficacy of postoperative continuous positive airway pressure to prevent pulmonary complications after roux-en-Y gastric bypass. J Gastrointest Surg. 2002;6(3):354–8.
26. Ramirez A, Lalor PF, Szomstein S, Rosenthal RJ. Continuous positive airway pressure in immediate postoperative period after laparoscopic roux-en-Y gastric bypass: is it safe? Surg Obes Relat Dis. 2009;5(5):544–6.
27. Weingarten TN, Kendrick ML, Swain JM, Liedl LM, Johnson CP, Schroeder DR, et al. Effects of CPAP on gastric pouch pressure after bariatric surgery. Obes Surg. 2011;21(12):1900–5.
28. Brill A-K. How to avoid interface problems in acute non-invasive ventilation. Breathe. 2014;10(3):230–42.

Non-invasive Ventilation in Solid Transplantation

Elena Giovanna Bignami

Contents

17.1 Kidney and Pancreas

Patients who are receiving (recipients) kidney, pancreas, and kidney-pancreas transplant usually have systemic comorbidities such as end-stage renal disease (ESRD) and diabetes which prone them more to postoperative complications. Kidney transplants account for about two-thirds of all solid organ transplants and offer to the patient an improved quality of life and overall survival at lower cost than kidney dialysis [1, 2].

Immunosuppressive therapy used to prevent graft rejection and in particular antilymphocyte globulin therapy leads to pulmonary complications. ARF is a relatively frequent cause of death in recipients with higher mortality rates in who develop opportunistic bacterial and fungal pneu-monia. Graft loss depends on reduction of blood flow, blood oxygenation or by use of toxic drugs. Severe ARF with lung infiltrates and consequent hypoxemia or septic shock and consequent hemo-dynamic instability lead to graft loss [1]. In order to efficacy treat ARF and avoid hypoxemia, ICU specialists can use NIV that is associated with decreased endotracheal intubation rate, fewer complications, and improved survival rate among immunocompromised patients [3]. However largely use of NIV in ARF-immunocompromised patient is questionable because of the rate failure reaches 50% and mortality increases when patients receive delayed invasive mechanical ventilation [3]. Patient characteristics favorable for treatment with non-invasive ventilation are: collaborative patient, intact neurological func-tion, capable of coordinating breathing with ven-tilator, moderate disease, teeth intact, capable of controlling oral and pulmonary secretions, mod-erate hypercapnia, moderate respiratory acidosis (pH > 7.20) [4].

E. G. Bignami (✉)

Anesthesiology, Critical Care and Pain Medicine Division, Department of Medicine and Surgery, University of Parma, Parma, Italy

e-mail: elenagiovanna.bignami@unipr.it

© The Author(s), under exclusive license to Springer Nature Switzerland AG 2023

G. Servillo, M. Vargas (eds.), *Non-invasive Mechanical Ventilation in Critical Care, Anesthesiology and Palliative Care*, https://doi.org/10.1007/978-3-031-36510-2_17

High-flow nasal cannula (HFNC) oxygen therapy delivers heated and fully humidified oxygen at high-flow rates through a nasal cannula reaching a maximum gas flow of 60 L/min and a constant fraction of inspired oxygen (FiO2) up to 100%. The device decreases respiratory rates with the use of high-flow oxygen, contributes to decrease the nasopharyngeal dead space and to generate a minimum of Positive End-Expiratory Pressure (PEEP), improves mucociliary function and secretion expectoration thanks to high grade of gas humidity thus to lower risk of respiratory infection [3].

HFNC is an alternative therapy to NIV in renal and pancreas transplant recipients with hypoxemic ARF secondary to severe pneumonia because of increased number of ventilator-free days at day 28, fewer complications, and no significant differences in intubation rate, length of ICU and hospital stays, and ICU and hospital mortalities compared with NIV treatment [2].

17.2　Liver

High immunosuppression level in liver-transplanted patients exposes them to nosocomial-acquired infections and consequent to increased morbidity, length of ICU stay, and mortality; these patients when mechanically ventilated are at high risk to develop ventilator-associated pneumonia (VAP) and persistence of an endotracheal tube is the single most important predisposing factor [5].

Although the real incidence in not clear, probably one-third of end-stage liver disease patients present a different grade of respiratory failure with abnormalities in gas exchange and widened Alveolar-arterial (A-a) oxygen gradient [6].

In end-stage liver disease patients, normal lung function is compromised by intrapulmonary shunting, ventilation/perfusion mismatch, hypoxic vasoconstrictor response failure, left ventricular failure, poor oxygen diffusion across dilated pulmonary capillaries, and interstitial edema of parenchyma. Low level of albumin in plasma leads to abdominal and pleural fluids' effusions that directly influence thorax compliance and induce restrictive disorder [7].

Neurological disorders and perioperative use of sedative drugs may affect the central regulation of breathing and cause hypoventilation; sometimes numerous failed attempts of weaning require prolonged tracheal intubation and mechanical ventilation [5].

In liver-transplanted patients is strongly recommended to achieve spontaneous ventilation as soon as possible in order to avoid ventilator-induced complications and negative hemodynamic effect on graft perfusion of high intrathoracic pressure [8]. Rapid extubation followed by prompt NIV application should be considered to shorten and accelerate the weaning process for recipients, reducing lung derecruitment through application of PEEP and Pressure Support (PS, a pressure delivered by the ventilator during the inspiratory phase). Liver transplant patients appear to tolerate NIV with mild (or no) sedation [5].

NIV enables both hypercapnic and hypoxic patients to improve faster, promoting cough and spontaneous expectoration of secretions because of less upper airways trauma compared to tracheal intubation and mechanical ventilation [9]. Continuous maintenance of a positive pressure in airways prevents alveoli collapse (atelectasis) and as largely demonstrated in heart failure patients reduces interstitial edema. In case of pre-existing heart failure, the application of an intra-thoracic positive pressure, reduces transmural ventricular pressure and preloads promoting better systolic function [10]. When patients need sedatives to facilitate rest, the use of NIV avoids eventually lung derecruitment and hypoxic nocturnal episodes [11].

High intrathoracic pressure reached during mechanical ventilation increases Inferior Vena Cava (IVC) pressure and so reduces the physiological gradient between IVC and Portal Vein; this condition can compromise intrahepatic blood flow and graft oxygenation [5, 8]. In order to avoid this complication, it is recommended to use ventilator pressure as low as possible; NIV obtains a more balanced intrathoracic hemodynamic than invasive technique also in hemodynamically unstable transplant patients [5, 10].

When patients are completely weaned by NIV in Pressure Support mode, usually a short and intermittent period of treatment with Continuous Positive Airway Pressure (CPAP) prevents alveoli collapsing during spontaneous ventilation and improves gas exchange [5]. The Helmet system efficacy delivers NIV treatment and reduces the side effects associated with prolonged use of a full facial mask, such as erythema, ulcerations on the nose and face, conjunctival irritation, discomfort on speaking, claustrophobia, sensation of air pressure, and air leaks. The helmet system is associated with a lower failure rate than a facial mask [12].

Respiratory failure in liver-transplanted patients is most of time related to intervening treatable events that respond to specific treatments: hemofiltration, pleural drainage, bronchial toilette, and abdominal drainage. NIV prolongs time during with patients can benefit from specific treatment supporting their pulmonary functions. In selected patients, NIV trial reduces the group whom requests reintubation. Patients who require reintubation are considered to be at high risk for ventilator-related complications [5, 13].

Also in children, atelectasis is common pulmonary complication especially after abdominal surgery. Recent evidences show that the need for reintubation due to pulmonary complications is significantly lower for liver-transplanted pediatric patients receiving NIV versus those not receiving NIV [13].

17.3 Lung

Some patients affected by end-stage lung diseases can receive lung transplant with great short- and medium-term survival rates; they have less than 2 years of life expectancy and no possibilities to improve their conditions only with medical therapy [4].

Joel Cooper performed the first successful single-lung transplant in 1983 and double-lung transplant in 1986.

Respiratory conditions that more frequently require transplant therapy are emphysema related to Chronic Obstructive Pulmonary Disease (COPD) with or without alpha-1-antitripsin deficit, Idiopathic Pulmonary Fibrosis (IPF), and others interstitial pneumopathy, cystic fibrosis or bronchiectasis, primary pulmonary hypertension [4, 14].

Nowadays, with more evidences in pediatric patients, it is recommended to perform double-lung transplant improving quality of life and long-term survival, despite greater perioperative morbidity and mortality [15]. Usually after surgery, double-lumen endotracheal tube is replaced with a single-lumen tube and the patient, admitted in ICU, is mechanically ventilated. Ventilatory parameters depend on recipient characteristic and single or double transplant; ICU specialists choose the Fraction of Inspired Oxygen (FiO_2) as low as possible to maintain an adequate peripherally oxygenation and Tidal Volume (TV) between 12 mL/Kg and 15 mL/Kg. Usually low levels of PEEP (5–8 cm H_2O) guarantee distal aeration [4]. In order to reduce hyperinflation of native lung in single-lung recipients, they had to better avoid PEEP and high TV. In most cases, recipients receive mechanical ventilation for about 24–48 h but in primary graft dysfunction, rejection or infection occurs, therapy must be prolonged [4].

Acute respiratory failure is the main cause of post-transplant mortality [16]. Although in postoperative period, numerous pulmonary complications can arise, special focus should be made on stenosis and dehiscence of airways, and vessels surgical anastomosis. In most cases of blood leakage, surgery is needed. Bronchial suture failure leads to air leakage in pleural cavity drained by thoracic tube; in this condition, either invasive or non-invasive positive pressure gets worse leakage preventing healing. If mostly of TV is lost through dehiscence, double-lumen tube needs to deliver optimal ventilation in the dehiscence-free lung and ventilation with the lowest possible pressure in the other lung [4].

The risk of barotrauma on airway sutures is particularly high within the first 2 weeks following lung transplantation especially in cases of insistent coughing or active expiration against the ventilator. Bronchus secretions' blind aspiration also damages anastomosis [17].

Fortunately, in clinical practice, many respiratory disorders following extubation may respond to specific interventions, such as fluid restriction, diuretics, bronchial toilette, cough induction, resolution of abdominal distension, and increased immunosuppression. NIV gives to the patients time, estimated in hours or days, to respond to specific treatments [17].

Use of NIV in lung-transplanted patient to treat respiratory failure significantly increases oxygenation and reduces reintubation, sepsis, and ICU mortality rate [4, 18].

Temporary graft dysfunction because of reperfusion injury is characterized by new radiographic findings and gas exchange abnormalities. The clinical picture includes pulmonary congestion, decreased lung compliance, diffuse or lobar patchy infiltrates, pulmonary hypertension, right ventricular failure, and respiratory fatigue. The aim of ventilatory management of this syndrome should be to maintain spontaneous breathing with active diaphragmatic movement. NIV triggered by spontaneous inspiratory effort leads to a greater distribution of inspired gas increasing the aeration of dysatelectatic areas [17].

NIV usually is well-tolerated, resolves atelectasis and lung infiltrates, treats extra vascular pulmonary fluid, and restores pulmonary volume, reducing dyspnea and respiratory effort [4]. Using of NIV increases time of slow and deep breathing pattern associated with better alveolar aeration [17].

Low sedation requested for NIV treatment allows an easier mobilization of patients from supine to prone or to sitting position; this approach recruits dorsal-basal areas of lungs and improves ventilation-perfusion ratio [4].

The incidence of pulmonary infections is higher in intubated recipients. The endotracheal tube may damage the tracheal mucosa and thereby increase the susceptibility to microorganism invasion, common features following ischemia-reperfusion damage to the graft. Consequently, withdrawal from invasive ventilation becomes mandatory for immunocompromised patients. In lungs recipients, strategies that could reduce period of invasive ventilation are epidural analgesia, early sitting position, physiotherapy, and non-invasive positive pressure ventilation by facial mask or helmet. Rapid extubation plus prompt NIV application is particularly suitable for lung recipients who do not completely fulfill the criteria for safe extubation. NIV preserves airway defense mechanisms and so plays an important role to prevent pneumonia in immunocompromised lung recipients. Endotracheal tube increases airway resistance and so causes extra work for inspiratory and expiratory muscles [17].

In a few double-lung transplanted patients, who presented respiratory failure after extubation, it was successfully used high-frequency percussive ventilation to avoid reintubation; it consists on delivering low volume at high rate that produces a more uniform gas exchange and better distal oxygenation. Other advantages of this time-cycled, limited pressure mode of ventilation are to facilitate elimination of secretion through vibrations and possible use with facemask or endotracheal tube. High frequencies (300–600 cycles per minute) improve oxygenation, while low frequencies (180–240) improve CO_2 elimination [19, 20].

Especially in patients suffering from heart failure, part of postoperative respiratory distress and dyspnea depends on lungs congestion and interstitial edema, NIV reduces extravascular lung water when diuretics alone are ineffective.

Physiotherapy represents an essential aspect of a lung transplant program; muscle weakness and stiff graft may increase patient effort reducing cooperation with physiotherapist. NIV reduces workload and oxygen consumption avoiding polypnea and CO_2 retention.

In postoperative period, NIV is also used to treat recipients with phrenic nerve injuries, in most cases caused by mediastinal dissection. Diaphragm reduction of movement or paralysis leads to atelectasis, pneumonia, hypoxemia, and hypoventilation. NIV may improve diaphragmatic electromyogram activity, decrease accessory muscle involvement, and reduce inspiratory muscle energy expenditure [17].

Hemodynamically unstable recipients treated with NIV have better Cardiac output than invasive mechanical ventilation due to lower ventilator pressure. In result of this, the consumption of inotropes and vasoactive drugs is lower.

The use of NIV is also been reported in the period before and after transplantation as a therapeutic option for chronic respiratory failure of multiple etiologies.

NIV nocturnal treatment prolongs life of patients waiting for transplant improving their quality of life and reducing frequency and severity of chronic lung disease exacerbations [11].

Chronic lung allograft dysfunction (CLAD) encompasses a range of pathologies that cause a transplanted lung to not achieve or maintain normal function. CLAD manifests as airflow restriction and/or obstruction and is predominantly a result of chronic rejection. Three distinct phenotypes of chronic rejection are now recognized: bronchiolitis obliterans, neutrophilic reversible allograft dysfunction, and restrictive allograft syndrome [21]. NIV seems to be a valuable treatment option for CLAD with favorable tolerability and security profiles [22].

17.4 Heart

Heart-transplanted patients receive strictly monitoring in Cardiac Surgery Intensive Care Unit (CSICU) in postoperative period because of some potential specific complications can occur [23]. Pulmonary complications are common with a prevalence from 5% to 20% and cause an increase in morbidity and mortality [24]. In most cases, heart recipients have comorbidities involving lungs because of close relationship in anatomy and function between the two organs [24]. Pulmonary hypertension development or worsening after transplant leads to acute right heart failure. Right Ventricle (RV) failure also depends on ischemia, arrhythmias or Primary Graft Dysfunction (PGD) [23]. Primary graft dysfunction is a life-threatening complication of heart transplantation that presents as left, right, or biventricular dysfunction occurring within the first 24 h of transplant surgery for which there is no identifiable secondary cause [25]. Management strategies to treat RV dysfunction and pulmonary hypertension focus on optimizing myocardial perfusion, preload, and contractility while reducing the pulmonary vascular resistance and its resulting RV afterload [23, 26]. Excessive pre-load leads to RV dilation reducing ejection fraction and performance. To reach adequate volemia is challenging and sometimes invasive monitoring is mandatory to dose correctly intravenous fluids and diuretics. Use of inodilator drugs increases myocardial contractility and reduces afterload and pulmonary hypertension [27, 28]. Although their administration may be limited by hypotension and vasopressor requirements. Inhaled nitric oxide or prostacyclin is also used to reduce pulmonary vascular resistance [28]. Pulmonary vascular resistance also depends on blood level of O_2 and CO_2, so correction of hypoxia and hypercapnia is essential to manage RV dysfunction and pulmonary hypertension. Hemogasanalysis and end-tidal CO_2 monitoring help to ensure the patient is not acidotic with optimal oxygenation and ventilation. Patients typically arrive in the CSICU intubated and on mechanical ventilation. In feasible conditions, patients should be extubated as soon as possible because of mechanical ventilation increases intrathoracic pressure and subsequently worsens pulmonary hypertension and also endotracheal tube increase risk of Ventilator-Associated Pneumoniae (VAP). If patients achieve hemodynamic stability but ventilator weaning is not safety because of hypoxia and hypercapnia risk, it is recommended to start a NIV trial in pressure support mode [23]. NIV should be considered in selected patients with postoperative acute respiratory failure to both prevent and treat acute respiratory failure following patient weaning from mechanical ventilation and tracheal extubation [29]. Prophylactic use of NIV reduced the rate of postoperative pulmonary complications in patients after cardiac surgery [24].

References

1. Canet E, Osman D, Lambert J, et al. Acute respiratory failure in kidney transplant recipients: a multicenter study. Crit Care. 2011;15(2):R91. https://doi.org/10.1186/cc10091.
2. Pretto EA, Biancofiore G, DeWolf A, Niemann C, Klinck PDS JR. Oxford textbook of transplant anaesthesia and critical care. Oxford University Press; 2015.
3. Tu G, He H, Yin K, Ju M, Zheng Y, Zhu D, Luo Z. High-flow nasal cannula versus noninvasive ven-

tilation for treatment of acute hypoxemic respiratory failure in renal transplant recipients. Transplant Proc. 2017;49:1325–30.

4. Tirado Conde G. Implications of non-invasive mechanical ventilation in lung transplantation. Old and new frontiers? Int J Pulm Respir Sci. 2017;1(1):IJOPRS.MS.ID.555555. https://doi.org/10.19080/ijoprs.2017.01.555555.

5. Feltracco P, Serra E, Barbieri S, Milevoj M, Salvaterra F, Marulli G, Ori C. Noninvasive ventilation in adult liver transplantation. Transplant Proc. 2008;40:1979–82.

6. Hourani JM, Bellamy PE, Tashkin DP, Batra P, Simmons MS. Pulmonary dysfunction in advanced liver disease: frequent occurrence of an abnormal diffusing capacity. Am J Med. 1991;90:693–700.

7. Battaglia SE, Pretto JJ, Irving LB, Jones RM, Angus PW. Resolution of gas exchange abnormalities and intrapulmonary shunting following liver transplantation. Hepatology. 1997;25:1228–32.

8. Celikel T, Sungur M, Ceyhan B, Karakurt S. Comparison of noninvasive positive pressure ventilation with standard medical therapy in hypercapnic acute respiratory failure. Chest. 1998;114:1636–42.

9. Hill NS. Noninvasive ventilation. Does it work, for whom, and how? Am Rev Respir Dis. 1993;147:1050–5.

10. Lenique F, Habis M, Lofaso F, Dubois-Randé JL, Harf A, Brochard L. Ventilatory and hemodynamic effects of continuous positive airway pressure in left heart failure. Am J Respir Crit Care Med. 1997;155:500–5.

11. Waldhorn RE. Nocturnal nasal intermittent positive pressure ventilation with bi-level positive airway pressure (BiPAP) in respiratory failure. Chest. 1992;101:516–21.

12. Antonelli M, Conti G, Pelosi P, Gregoretti C, Pennisi MA, Costa R, Severgnini P, Chiaranda M, Proietti R. New treatment of acute hypoxemic respiratory failure: noninvasive pressure support ventilation delivered by helmet--a pilot controlled trial. Crit Care Med. 2002;30:602–8.

13. Murase K, Chihara Y, Takahashi K, Okamoto S, Segawa H, Fukuda K, Tanaka K, Uemoto S, Mishima M, Chin K. Use of noninvasive ventilation for pediatric patients after liver transplantation: decrease in the need for reintubation. Liver Transplant. 2012;18:1217–25.

14. Group TLT. Unilateral lung transplantation for pulmonary fibrosis. N Engl J Med. 1986;314:1140–5.

15. Force SD, Kilgo P, Neujahr DC, Pelaez A, Pickens A, Fernandez FG, Miller DL, Lawrence C. Bilateral lung transplantation offers better long-term survival, compared with single-lung transplantation, for younger patients with idiopathic pulmonary fibrosis. Ann Thorac Surg. 2011;91:244–9.

16. Cooper JD, Patterson GA, Trulock EP. Results of single and bilateral lung transplantation in 131 consecutive recipients. Washington university lung transplant group. J Thorac Cardiovasc Surg. 1994;107:460–1.

17. Feltracco P, Serra E, Barbieri S, Milevoj M, Furnari M, Rizzi S, Rea F, Marulli G, Ori C. Noninvasive ventilation in postoperative care of lung transplant recipients. Transplant Proc. 2009;41:1339–44.

18. Rocco M, Conti G, Antonelli M, Bufi M, Costa MG, Alampi D, Ruberto F, Stazi GV, Pietropaoli P. Noninvasive pressure support ventilation in patients with acute respiratory failure after bilateral lung transplantation. Intensive Care Med. 2001;27:1622–6.

19. Feltracco P, Serra E, Barbieri S, Milevoj M, Michieletto E, Carollo C, Rea F, Zanus G, Boetto R, Ori C. Noninvasive high-frequency percussive ventilation in the prone position after lung transplantation. Transplant Proc. 2012;44:2016–21.

20. Lucangelo U, Fontanesi L, Antonaglia V, Pellis T, Berlot G, Liguori G, Bird FM, Gullo A. High-frequency percussive ventilation (HFPV). Principles and technique. Minerva Anestesiol. 2003;69.:841–8:848–51.

21. Gauthier JM, Hachem RR, Kreisel D. Update on chronic lung allograft dysfunction. Curr Transplant Rep. 2016;3:185–91.

22. Magalhães AR, Moreira I, Caldeira V, Sá T, Borba A, Calvinho P, Semedo L, Cardoso J, Fragata J. Non-invasive ventilation post lung transplantation in a home setting. Eur Respir J. 2020;56:403.

23. Rabin J, Kaczorowski DJ. Perioperative management of the cardiac transplant recipient. Crit Care Clin. 2019;35:45–60.

24. Liu Q, Shan M, Liu J, Cui L, Lan C. Prophylactic noninvasive ventilation versus conventional care in patients after cardiac surgery. J Surg Res. 2020;246:384–94.

25. Chew HC, Kumarasinghe G, Iyer A, et al. Primary graft dysfunction after heart transplantation. Curr Transplant Rep. 2014;1:257–65.

26. Vega E, Schroder J, Nicoara A. Postoperative management of heart transplantation patients. Best Pract Res Clin Anaesthesiol. 2017;31:201–13.

27. Simsch O, Gromann T, Knosalla C, Hübler M, HL RH. No title the intensive care management of patients following heart transplantation at the Deutsches Herzzentrum Berlin. Appl Cardiopulm Pathophysiol. 2011;15:230–40.

28. De Wet CJ, Affleck DG, Jacobsohn E, Avidan MS, Tymkew H, Hill LL, Zanaboni PB, Moazami N, Smith JR. Inhaled prostacyclin is safe, effective, and affordable in patients with pulmonary hypertension, right heart dysfunction, and refractory hypoxemia after cardiothoracic surgery. J Thorac Cardiovasc Surg. 2004;127:1058–67.

29. Guarracino F, Ambrosino N. Non invasive ventilation in cardio-surgical patients. Minerva Anestesiol. 2011;77:734–41.

Non-invasive Positive Pressure Ventilation in Patients Undergoing Lung Resection Surgery

Salvatore Lucio Cutuli, Joel Vargas, Simone Carelli, Eloisa Sofia Tanzarella, Gabriele Pintaudi, Domenico Luca Grieco, and Gennaro De Pascale

Contents

S. L. Cutuli · J. Vargas · S. Carelli · E. S. Tanzarella ·
G. Pintaudi · D. L. Grieco
Dipartimento di Scienze dell' Emergenza,
Anestesiologiche e della Rianimazione, Fondazione
Policlinico Universitario A. Gemelli IRCCS,
Rome, Italy
e-mail: salvatorelucio.cutuli@policlinicogemelli.it;
joel.vargas@policlinicogemelli.it;
simone.carelli@policlinicogemelli.it;
eloisasofia.tanzarella@policlinicogemelli.it;
gabriele.pintaudi@policlinicogemelli.it;
domenicoluca.grieco@policlinicogemelli.it

G. De Pascale (✉)
Dipartimento di Scienze dell' Emergenza,
Anestesiologiche e della Rianimazione, Fondazione
Policlinico Universitario A. Gemelli IRCCS,
Rome, Italy

Facoltà di medicina e chirurgia "A. Gemelli",
Università Cattolica del Sacro Cuore, Rome, Italy
e-mail: gennaro.depascale@policlinicogemelli.it

© The Author(s), under exclusive license to Springer Nature Switzerland AG 2023
G. Servillo, M. Vargas (eds.), *Non-invasive Mechanical Ventilation in Critical Care, Anesthesiology and Palliative Care*, https://doi.org/10.1007/978-3-031-36510-2_18

18.1 Introduction

Lung resection surgery has been widely performed in daily clinical practise and represents a major risk factor for postoperative pulmonary complications (PPCs) [1], mainly related to both patient's comorbidities and surgical aggression. In this setting, acute respiratory failure (ARF) has been considered the most severe life-threatening PPC, leading to re-intubation and invasive mechanical ventilation. On top of that, these interventions were demonstrated to increase the risk of worse clinical outcomes via the development of bronchial stump disruption, broncho-pleural fistula, persistent air leakage, and pulmonary infection [2].

Severe postoperative pulmonary complications may require admission to the Intensive Care Unit (ICU) and prolong hospital length of stay, with significant impact on quality of life and resource expenditure. Accordingly, several non-invasive respiratory support strategies [3] have been tested with the aim to prevent (prophylactic treatment) and early manage (curative treatment) PPCs [4], in order to improve patient-centred clinical outcomes.

In this chapter. we provided an overview of the epidemiology and pathophysiology of PPCs in patients undergoing lung resection surgery. Furthermore, we discussed the role of non-invasive respiratory support strategies in this setting [3], with a special focus on safety and effectiveness of high flow nasal cannula (HFNC), non-invasive positive pressure ventilation (NPPV), and continuous positive airway pressure (CPAP) compared with low flow oxygen therapy.

18.2 Epidemiology of Postoperative Pulmonary Complications After Lung Resection Surgery

In recent years, lung resection surgery has been widely implemented due to its best performance of diagnostic criteria for early identification of pulmonary cancer and technological discoveries [5] that have made possible this intervention even in extreme clinical conditions (e.g. advanced disease and high-risk patients). Although these improvements have carried significant benefits on patient-centred clinical outcomes, PPCs remain the leading cause of morbidity and mortality in this clinical setting [6]. PPCs have been broadly defined as "any pulmonary abnormality occurring in the postoperative period that produces identifiable disease or dysfunction which is clinically significant and adversely affects the clinical course" [7], and occur in 30% of patients (ranging from 7% to 49%), accounting for the 2–5% of in-hospital deaths [8]. In most of the cases, PPCs develop in the immediate postoperative period (hours and days) and are rarely described later on (weeks). Epidemiological studies showed that pre-operative patient functional status (age, independence in daily common activities, cardiovascular and pulmonary comorbidities, organ function reserve, previous chemotherapy, and/or radiation), surgical invasiveness [7, 8], and perioperative complications (blood loss, transfusion of blood products, excessive positive fluid balance and need for re-intervention) [9] play a role of paramount importance to determine the development of PPCs after lung resection surgery. Potentially, PPCs may involve any anatomical district of the thorax (airways, lungs, vessels, pleural serous, and diaphragm) and are mainly represented by persistent air leak (50%), atelectasis, and pneumonia (10–20%) [10, 11]. Specifically, air leaks are particularly frequent in patients with chronic lung diseases (emphysema or fibrosis) or pleural adhesions; atelectasis mostly occur after right upper lobectomy [10, 12]; pneumonia is favoured by open surgery, older age, chronic obstruction pulmonary disease (COPD), diabetes, history of previous pneumonia, atelectasis, and prolonged mechanical ventilation [13]. Although ARF accounts for 3% of PPCs and its incidence is directly associated with the invasiveness of surgery [2, 14], being more frequent after pneumonectomy than lobectomy or sub-lobar resection, this complication is burdened by the highest risk of mortality, which ranges between 52% and 65% [14]. Other PPCs like empyema (1%), haemothorax (0.3%), and direct diaphragmatic injury are quite rare, even if non-surgical diaphragmatic dysfunction has been recently described as a frequent condition after thoracic surgery [15]. Unfortunately, well-conducted multicentre epidemiologic studies and homogeneous diagnostic criteria for PPCs after lung resection surgery are lacking and these phenomena warrant further attention by the scientific community in order to best define their burden.

Finally, non-surgical diaphragmatic dysfunction is quite common after thoracic surgery and may be the result of paralysis, prolonged mechanical ventilation, and inflammation that favour muscle atrophy [16]. Also, non-surgical diaphragmatic dysfunction represents a significant risk factor for atelectasis, pneumonia, and ARF [16].

18.3 Pathophysiology of Postoperative Pulmonary Complications After Lung Resection Surgery

Several pathophysiological pathways may lead to the development of PPCs, which commonly end up with dyspnoea and impaired gas exchange (hypoxemia and hypercapnia). These clinical signs are caused by the detrimental effect of PPCs on ventilation/perfusion ratio, especially in patients with baseline and surgery-induced reduction of functional residual capacity of the lung [15].

As a matter of fact, persistent air leaks may be caused by pleural adhesions or dysfunctional lung parenchyma that cause heterogenous distribution of transpulmonary pression and impair wound healing. Furthermore, many similar features explain the pathophysiology of atelectasis and pneumonia that are mainly caused by hypoventilation and retained secretions. Both conditions result from diaphragmatic and thoraco-abdominal muscle dysfunction, suboptimal pain control, or excessive sedatives administration that limit inspiratory pulmonary expansion and cough reflex, with increased risk of gastric content aspiration. Moreover, comorbidities like COPD play a role of paramount importance due to concurrent sarcopenia and increased production of bronchial secretions. On the other hand, ARF and, specifically, Acute Respiratory Distress Syndrome (ARDS), may be caused by the inflammatory burst induced by extensive lung resection surgery, pneumonia, and sepsis, leading to non-cardiogenic pulmonary oedema. On the contrary, haemothorax is frequently caused by surgical factors and, quite rarely, by patients-related haemostasis disorders, while empyema represents a complication of pneumonia in most of the cases.

18.4 Role of Non-invasive Respiratory Support Strategies After Lung Resection Surgery

18.4.1 High Flow Nasal Cannula Oxygen Therapy

Effectiveness and safety of HFNC compared with low flow oxygen therapy to prevent postoperative pulmonary complication in patients undergoing lung resection surgery were investigated by small physiological studies. Specifically, HFNC was demonstrated to effectively improve oxygenation [17], reintubation [17] and length of hospital stay [18], although it had no impact on postoperative pulmonary complications [17, 19, 20]. However, a recent review and meta-analysis of the evidence available in this field [21] found that HFNC compared with low flow oxygen therapy in patients who underwent cardiac or thoracic surgery was associated with significantly lower reintubation rate (moderate certainty) and decreased need to escalate respiratory support (very low certainty), although it had no effect on mortality, incidence of postoperative hypoxia, ICU, and hospital length of stay. Sensitivity analysis showed that HFNC may prevent respiratory failure in specific patient population (obese and at high risk of postoperative respiratory complications), for whom current guidelines [21] recommended its use in the immediate postoperative period (conditional recommendation, moderate certainty of evidence) while suggested against its prophylactic use in other postsurgical patients. No randomised clinical studies have investigated the effectiveness of HFNC compared to low flow oxygen therapy to treat postoperative pulmonary complications after lung resection surgery.

18.4.2 Non-invasive Positive Pressure Ventilation and Continuous Positive Airway Pressure

Effectiveness and safety of NPPV compared with low flow oxygen therapy in patients undergoing lung resection surgery who developed postoperative ARF was initially investigated in 48 patients, showing that NPPV reduced the need for re-intubation and hospital mortality compared with standard practise [22]. On the other hand, small physiological studies showed that the prophylactic use of NPPV compared with low flow oxygen therapy was demonstrated to be safe and effective to improve blood oxygenation [23] and pulmonary function [24, 25], although these results were not replicated in a larger study on 349 patients with Chronic Obstructive Pulmonary Disease (COPD) who received this intervention more than 4 h after extubation [26]. According to these results, NPPV should be delivered to selected patient population [3], as soon as extubation (prophylactic treatment) or ARF (curative treatment) [27] occur, under the supervision of experienced personnel and adequate monitoring of therapy failure [3].

Furthermore, recent evidence showed that prophylactic continuous positive airway pressure (CPAP) applied immediately after extubation compared with low flow oxygen therapy may play a role to improving oxygenation [28], reducing postoperative atelectasis and pneumonia with no increased risk of air leaks and pneumothorax [29]. No randomised clinical studies have investigated the effectiveness of CPAP compared to low flow oxygen therapy to treat postoperative complications after lung resection surgery.

18.4.3 High Flow Nasal Cannula Oxygen Therapy Vs Non-invasive Positive Pressure Ventilation

Only one trial [30] compared HFNC oxygen therapy and NPPV in 830 patients with or at risk for ARF after cardiothoracic surgery (only 64 patients underwent lung resection) and found that there was no difference on treatment failure between these non-invasive respiratory support strategies. Moreover, secondary outcomes revealed that NPPV was more effective to improve hypoxemia compared to HFNC oxygen therapy, although the former was associated with major proportion of skin breakdown during the first 2 days.

18.5 Conclusions

Patients undergoing lung resection surgery are at risk of postoperative pulmonary complications, which development results from the interplay between comorbidities and surgical characteristics. Although an increasing amount of evidence supports the safety of postoperative HFNC, NPPV, and CPAP in this setting and each strategy may play a potential role to revert some pathophysiological pathways that sustain PPCs, the heterogeneity among patient populations, surgery characteristics, and indications for these therapies (prophylactic vs curative) do not allow to draw final conclusions on their effectiveness and superiority of one support over another. Accordingly, further research is warranted in this field, with the aim to place a role for each non-invasive respiratory support strategy in order to best match patient's need and improve related clinical outcomes.

References

1. Kirsh M, Rotman H, Behrendt D, Orringer M, Sloan H. Complications of pulmonary resection. Ann Thorac Surg. 1975;20(2):215–36.
2. Kutlu C, Williams E, Evans T, Pastorino U, Goldstraw P. Acute lung injury and acute respiratory distress syndrome after pulmonary resection. Ann Thorac Surg. 2000;69(2):376–80.
3. Leone M, Einav S, Chiumello D, Constantin J, Robertis ED, Md A, Gregoretti C, Jaber S, Maggiore S, Pelosi P, et al. Noninvasive respiratory support in the hypoxaemic peri-operative/periprocedural patient: a joint ESA/ESICM guideline. Intensive Care Med. 2020;46(4):697–713.
4. Jaber S, Antonelli M. Preventive or curative postoperative noninvasive ventilation after thoracic surgery: still a grey zone? Intensive Care Med. 2014;40(2):280–3.

5. Onugha O, Ivey R, McKenna R. Novel techniques and approaches to minimally invasive thoracic surgery. Surg Technol Int. 2017;30:231–5.

6. Hernández MG, Valentín N, Alvarado IR, Gago MF, Simó GV, López MJ. Changes in the risk of mortality and morbidity after lung resection in the last 20 years. Arch Bronconeumol (Engl Ed). 2020;56(1):23–7.

7. Agostini P, Cieslik H, Rathinam S, Bishay E, Kalkat M, Rajesh P, Steyn R, Singh S, Naidu B. Postoperative pulmonary complications following thoracic surgery: are there any modifiable risk factors? Thorax. 2010;65(9):815–8.

8. Stéphan F, Boucheseiche S, Hollande J, Flahault A, Cheffi A, Bazelly B, Bonnet F. Pulmonary complications following lung resection: a comprehensive analysis of incidence and possible risk factors. Chest. 2000;118(5):1263–70.

9. Miserocchi G, Beretta E, Rivolta I. Respiratory mechanics and fluid dynamics after lung resection surgery. Thorac Surg Clin. 2010;20(3):345–57.

10. Stolz A, Schutzner J, Lischke R, Simonek J, Harustiak T, Pafko P. Predictors of atelectasis after pulmonary lobectomy. Surg Today. 2008;38(11):987–92.

11. Schussler O, Alifano M, Dermine H, Strano S, Casetta A, Sepulveda S, Chafik A, Coignard S, Rabbat A, Regnard J. Postoperative pneumonia after major lung resection. Am J Respir Crit Care Med. 2006;173(10):1161–9.

12. Korst R, Humphrey C. Complete lobar collapse following pulmonary lobectomy. Its incidence, predisposing factors, and clinical ramifications. Chest. 1997;111(5):1285–9.

13. Simonsen D, Søgaard M, Bozi I, Horsburgh C, Thomsen R. Risk factors for postoperative pneumonia after lung cancer surgery and impact of pneumonia on survival. Respir Med. 2015;109(10):1340–6.

14. Dulu A, Pastores S, Park B, Riedel E, Rusch V, Halpern N. Prevalence and mortality of acute lung injury and ARDS after lung resection. Chest. 2006;130(1):73–8.

15. Thorpe A, Rodrigues J, Kavanagh J, Batchelor T, Lyen S. Postoperative complications of pulmonary resection. Clin Radiol. 2020;75(11):876.e871–6.

16. McCool F, Tzelepis G. Dysfunction of the diaphragm. N Engl J Med. 2012;366(10):932–42.

17. Yu Y, Qian X, Liu C, Zhu C. Effect of high-flow nasal cannula versus conventional oxygen therapy for patients with thoracoscopic lobectomy after extubation. Can Respir J. 2017;2017:7894631.

18. Ansari B, Hogan M, Collier T, Baddeley R, Scarci M, Coonar A, Bottrill F, Martinez G, Klein A. A randomized controlled trial of high-flow nasal oxygen (optiflow) as part of an enhanced recovery program after lung resection surgery. Ann Thorac Surg. 2016;101(2):459–64.

19. Brainard J, Scott B, Sullivan B, Fernandez-Bustamante A, Piccoli J, Gebbink M, Bartels K. Heated humidified high-flow nasal cannula oxygen after thoracic surgery - a randomized prospective clinical pilot trial. J Crit Care. 2017;40:225–8.

20. Pennisi M, Bello G, Congedo M, Montini L, Nachira D, Ferretti G, Meacci E, Gualtieri E, Pascale GD, Grieco D, et al. Early nasal high-flow versus venturi mask oxygen therapy after lung resection: a randomized trial. Crit Care. 2019;23(1):68.

21. Rochwerg B, Einav S, Chaudhuri D, Mancebo J, Mauri T, Helviz Y, Goligher E, Jaber S, Ricard J, Rittayamai N, et al. The role for high flow nasal cannula as a respiratory support strategy in adults: a clinical practice guideline. Intensive Care Med. 2020;46(12):2226–37.

22. Auriant I, Jallot A, Hervé P, Cerrina J, Ladurie FLR, Fournier J, Lescot B, Parquin F. Noninvasive ventilation reduces mortality in acute respiratory failure following lung resection. Am J Respir Crit Care Med. 2001;164(7):1231–5.

23. Aguiló R, Togores B, Pons S, Rubí M, Barbé F, Agustí A. Noninvasive ventilatory support after lung resectional surgery. Chest. 1997;112(1):117–21.

24. Perrin C, Jullien V, Vénissac N, Berthier F, Padovani B, Guillot F, Coussement A, Mouroux J. Prophylactic use of noninvasive ventilation in patients undergoing lung resectional surgery. Respir Med. 2007;101(7):1572–8.

25. Liao G, Chen R, He J. Prophylactic use of noninvasive positive pressure ventilation in post-thoracic surgery patients: a prospective randomized control study. J Thorac Dis. 2010;2(4):205–9.

26. Lorut C, Lefebvre A, Planquette B, Quinquis L, Clavier H, Santelmo N, Hanna H, Bellenot F, Regnard J, Riquet M, et al. Early postoperative prophylactic noninvasive ventilation after major lung resection in COPD patients: a randomized controlled trial. Intensive Care Med. 2014;40(2):220–7.

27. Rochwerg B, Brochard L, Elliott M, Hess D, Hill N, Nava S, Navalesi P, Committee MOTS, Antonelli M, Brozek J, et al. Official ERS/ATS clinical practice guidelines: noninvasive ventilation for acute respiratory failure. Eur Respir J. 2017;50(2):1602426.

28. Garutti I, Puente-Maestu L, Laso J, Sevilla R, Ferrando A, Frias I, Reyes A, Ojeda E, Gónzalez-Aragoneses F. Comparison of gas exchange after lung resection with a boussignac CPAP or venturi mask. Br J Anaesth. 2014;112(5):929–35.

29. Puente-Maestú L, López E, Sayas J, Alday E, Planas A, Parise D, Martínez-Borja M, Garutti I. Group Ps: the effect of immediate postoperative boussignac CPAP on adverse pulmonary events after thoracic surgery: a multicentre, randomised controlled trial. Eur J Anaesthesiol. 2021;38(2):164–70.

30. Stéphan F, Barrucand B, Petit P, Rézaiguia-Delclaux S, Médard A, Delannoy B, Cosserant B, Flicoteaux G, Imbert A, Pilorge C, et al. High-flow nasal oxygen vs noninvasive positive airway pressure in hypoxemic patients after cardiothoracic surgery: a randomized clinical trial. JAMA. 2015;313(23):2331–9.

Part VI

Non-invasive Ventilation Analgesia and Sedation

Sedation and Analgesia During Non-invasive Ventilation in Intensive Care

19

A. Marra, P. P. Pandharipande, and Giuseppe Servillo

Content

Non-invasive ventilation (NIV) is currently one of the most commonly used support methods in hypoxemic and hypercapnic acute respiratory failure (ARF). With advancing technology and increasing experience, indications for NIV are getting broader and more severe patients are treated with NIV. Success of NIV is strongly dependent on the patient's degree of tolerance and collaboration during ventilation. One of the most frequent causes of premature interruption of

A. Marra (✉)
Department of Neurosciences, Reproductive and Odontostomatological Sciences, University of Naples "Federico II", Naples, Italy

Critical Illness, Brain Dysfunction, and Survivorship (CIBS) Center, Vanderbilt University School of Medicine, Nashville, TN, USA

P. P. Pandharipande
Critical Illness, Brain Dysfunction, and Survivorship (CIBS) Center, Vanderbilt University School of Medicine, Nashville, TN, USA

Department of Anesthesiology, Division of Critical Care Medicine, Vanderbilt University School of Medicine, Nashville, TN, USA

G. Servillo
Department of Neurosciences, Reproductive and Odontostomatological Sciences, University of Naples "Federico II", Naples, Italy

the NIV is mask intolerance due to pain, discomfort, or claustrophobia [1, 2]. Relative contraindications to NIV are delirium and agitation [3]. Judicious sedation may play a crucial role in improving patient's tolerance in selected cases at risk of endotracheal intubation due to NIV failure.

Although intolerance is commonly perceived as an important reason for NIV failure that should respond to sedation and analgesia, Muriel et al. [4] found that sedation and analgesia were used in about 20% of patients using NIV, confirming the results of a survey performed in North America and Europe [5]. Therefore, the large majority of patients (approximately 80%) treated with NIV for acute respiratory failure do not receive any form of sedation and yet tolerate NIV and usually succeed with it [4, 6]. There are several reasons that could be related to poor NIV acceptance and any decision to resort to sedation must be taken as the last stage in a careful evaluation of the causes of actual or pending failure. The patient acceptance varies according to the type of mask that is used, as it is greatest with the least constricting interfaces, such as the helmet, and declines with more intrusive forms of a mask. Also, the assisted ventilation pattern can influence patient compliance (e.g., bilevel positive airways pressure often produces a need for sedation whereas spontaneous breathing models such as continuous positive airways pressure seldom require such interventions) [7].

Despite numerous non-pharmacological strategies may be employed to avert NIV failure, some patients remain intolerant and uncooperative with a poor patient–ventilator synchrony. Even though sedation is not mandatory for NIV, it may help under these circumstances, in the attempt to reverse the situation may be worthwhile before the intubation.

The use of sedation in patients receiving respiratory support from NIV is an area of critical and intensive care medicine where there are limited, if any, robust data to guide the development of best practice and where local custom appears to exert a strong influence on patterns of care. Any decision to start sedation must be taken as the last stage in a careful evaluation of the causes of discomfort [7] (Fig. 19.1).

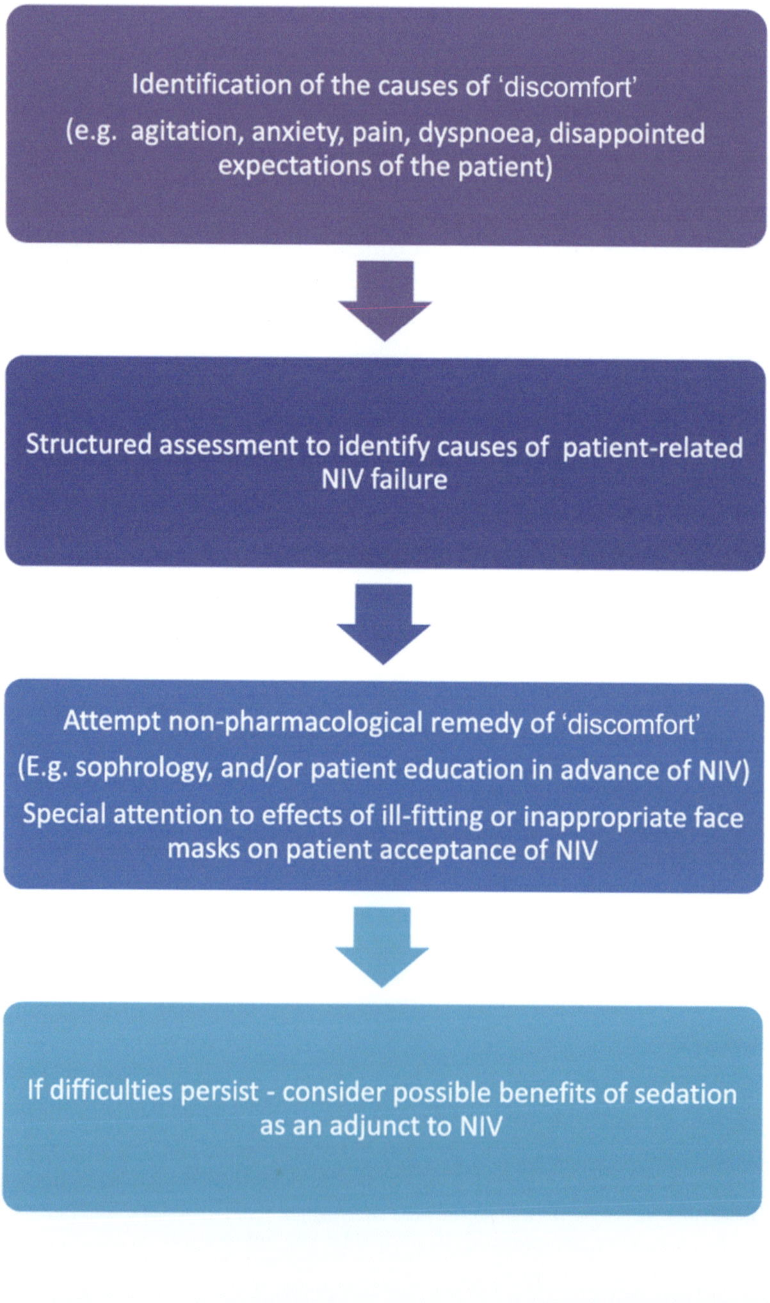

Fig. 19.1 Clinical reasoning pathway for the use of sedation in NIV (Longrois et al. [7])

Identification of the causes of 'discomfort'

(e.g. agitation, anxiety, pain, dyspnoea, disappointed expectations of the patient)

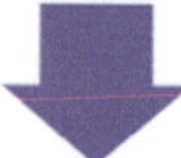

Structured assessment to identify causes of patient-related NIV failure

Attempt non-pharmacological remedy of 'discomfort'

(E.g. sophrology, and/or patient education in advance of NIV)

Special attention to effects of ill-fitting or inappropriate face masks on patient acceptance of NIV

If difficulties persist - consider possible benefits of sedation as an adjunct to NIV

The goals of sedation for a cooperative patient in the ICU are to provide analgesia and comfort, preserve day/night cycles (including natural sleep), and avoid nuisances such as ambient light and noise. Additional goals include hemodynamic stability, preservation of metabolic homeostasis, muscular relaxation, preservation of diaphragmatic function, and attenuation of the stress/immune response, as well as considerations such as programmed withdrawal from sedation: they should be no different during NIV [7]. In addition, sedation during NIV should be performed with no/minimal respiratory depression and no/minimal impairment of the upper airway [7], in a setting where patients can be monitored continuously. Several sedation scales are available and may be helpful in ensuring that the level of sedation is minimized and the PAD guidelines recommend the use of the Richmond Agitation-Sedation Scale (RASS) and the Riker Sedation-Agitation Scale (SAS) [8, 9].

The ideal sedative drug during NIV should have a rapid onset, a predictable duration of action, a constant half-life time, a no impact on the hemodynamic and respiratory drive, an organ-independent metabolism, a minimal drug interaction, and, finally, a low cost.

Benzodiazepines and opioids have effects on airways patency and respiratory drive the timing. Moreover, sometimes it could also be difficult to titrate their pharmacologic effects because they may accumulate with repeated dosing. Benzodiazepines may also be associated with a greater risk of delirium and cognitive impairment [10]. A continuous infusion of opiates did not reduce respiratory drive but showed detrimental effects on respiratory timing both when airway occlusion pressure at 0.1 s (P0.1) was assessed [11, 12] or when electrical activity of the diaphragm (EAdi) was directly measured [13].

Propofol has also been shown to increase the collapsibility of the upper airway in a dose/concentration-dependent manner [7]. Measuring the EAdi, Vaschetto et al. showed in intubated patients that propofol significantly interferes with the patient-ventilator synchrony in pressure support ventilation (PSV) at doses producing deep sedation. Both during PSV and neurally adjusted ventilator assistance (NAVA), propofol reduced neural drive and effort, while not significantly affecting respiratory timing [14]. Clouzeau et al. evaluated, in a population of ten patients with acute respiratory failure at risk of NIV failure due to poor tolerance, the safety of target-controlled infusion technique (TCI) propofol infusion for sedation [15]. In this study, NIV under TCI of propofol improved arterial blood gas analyses: mean PF increased from 167 ± 68 pre-session to 195 ± 68 post-session ($p < 0.05$), mean PaCO2 decreased from 57.8 ± 15.3 to 49 ± 9.8 mmHg ($p < 0.05$) and mean pH increased from 7.36 ± 0.04 to 7.4 ± 0.03 ($p < 0.05$). Within the limits of a pilot study, TCI of propofol seems to be safe and effective for the treatment of NIV failure due to low tolerance [15].

Among the sedative drugs, dexmedetomidine, an alpha 2 adrenoreceptor agonist, seems to have a most suitable overall pharmacological profile and could be of interest in patients receiving NIV. Dexmedetomidine provides sedation and analgesia with attenuation of the stress response with no significant respiratory depression and has no direct effects on the patency of the upper airways. Continuous intravenous infusion should start at a dose between 0.2 mg/kg/h and 1.4 mg/kg/h, and no loading dose should be administered. When used as adjunct therapy it may reduce requirements for opioids and other sedatives and so reduce the likelihood of opioid-induced compromise of the upper airways. There are only a few studies regarding the use of dexmedetomidine during NIV, with reduced sample size and with conflicting results. Senoglu et al. tested the sedative profile and adverse events of dexmedetomidine against midazolam in an ICU population of patients undergoing NIV for ARF secondary to COPD exacerbation [16]. In both groups, sedation was targeted to achieve either a score 2–3 RASS or a score 3/4 Riker sedation-agitation scale or a bispectral index level > 85. No serious cardiovascular adverse events or NIV failures were documented. However, during the sedation induction period, heart rate and blood pressure were significantly lower in the group treated with dexmedetomidine (incidence of bradycardia: 18.2% vs. 0, $p = 0.016$). In terms of respiratory frequency and gas exchanges, no significative differences were found between the two groups [17]. Though no patient experienced NIV failure during the study period, compared to midazolam, dexmedetomidine required fewer dosing adjustments to maintain adequate sedation ($p < 0.01$) [16]. This study, however, considers only the first 24 h of NIV and does not provide valuable information on any outcome variable [16]. Huang et al. randomized 62 hypoxemic patients with acute pulmonary edema refusing to continue the NIV due to high discomfort and marked agitation into two groups of treatment: midazolam or dexmedetomidine [17]. This study did not report serious adverse events, and none of the patients interrupted the study protocol; bradycardia occurred more with dexmedetomidine (18.2% vs. 0, $p = 0.016$). The rate of failure (e.g. endotracheal intubation) was overall 32%. In the dexmedetomidine group of patients, NIV failure was lower (21%) than in the midazolam group (45%), $p = 0.043$. In addition, dexmedetomidine led to a more desired level of awake sedation, shortened the duration of mechanical ventilation and the length of ICU stay. Healthcare-associated infections were reduced, apparently because with dexmedetomidine no blunting of the cough reflex was observed [17]. Devlin et al. enrolled 33 adult patients with ARF within 8 h after starting NIV and divided them into two groups to receive dexmedetomidine (preventive approach) or placebo up to 72 h [18]. Patients with agitation or pain could also receive a bolus of midazolam or fentanyl by intravenous administration. Intravenous dexmedetomidine infusion starting soon after NIV initiation does not maintain adequate levels of sedation and does not improve NIV tolerance. The authors attested that in a population of subjects undergoing NIV treatment, of which only one-third showed at baseline signs of NIV intolerance, a routine and early dexmedetomidine infusion does not bring any advantage over an intermittent bolus of fentanyl and midazolam. In fact, there was no significative difference in the prevention of agitation and delirium, no reduction in NIV failure rate, or any improvement in patient/nursing staff comfort [18]. The study conducted by Shutes et al. retrospectively reviewed the chart of the patients who received dexmedetomidine infusion for >24 h and their discontinuation pattern and its relation with hemodynamics of the patients and withdrawal [19]. The study found that the dexmedetomidine sedation was having a predictive hemodynamic effect. The cumulative dose was associated with withdrawal, but symptoms were manageable with short-term enteral clonidine. Venkatraman et al. also conducted a retrospective evaluation including pediatric patients who received NIV and dexmedetomidine infusion within 48 h of ICU admission. The study found the dexmedetomidine infusion as the single continuous sedative was effective; however, dose titration was required to get rid of mild cardiorespiratory events [20]. Piastra et al. also performed one retrospective analysis of data from 40 pediatric group patients who were receiving NIV for ARF [21]. They analyzed the effectiveness of dexmedetomidine as infusion sedative and found that early dexmedetomidine infusion in such patients was safe and effective in reducing patient–ventilator synchronization and permitting lung recruitment. Ni et al. also conducted one retrospective study including 80 adult patients [22]. They evaluated the effect of sedation and/or analgesia as rescue treatment during NIV in the patients with interface intolerance after extubation and found that sedation and/or analgesia treatment can decrease the rate of NIV failure. The study also found decreased hospital mortality rate and ICU LOS in patients who received analgesia and/or sedation.

Haloperidol is a D2 receptor antagonist. Blockade of D2 receptors may result in improvement of hallucination and delusions. The use of haloperidol can also reduce the need for sedative and analgesic drugs in ventilated patients. Haloperidol has a number of side effects, including extrapyramidal manifestations and rarely neuroleptic malignant syndrome but the most dangerous adverse effect is prolongation of the corrected QT (QTc) interval which can precipitate fatal arrhythmias.

Ketamine does not cause respiratory depression at doses given for analgesia or procedural sedation. Furthermore, it decreases airway resistance, improves dynamic compliance, and preserves functional residual capacity, minute ventilation, and tidal volume, while retaining protective pharyngeal and laryngeal reflexes. Ketamine can produce hypersalivation and emergence reactions. Because of its effects on the sympathetic nervous system, ketamine should not be used in decompensated heart failure (typically cardiogenic pulmonary edema in the context of NIV). Despite its advantages, there is a relatively poor literature concerning the use of ketamine during NIV.

There is limited published data available regarding delirium in NIV. From this limited data, delirium is associated with NIV failure and the risk of this is 112% more than that in nondelirious patients [23]. Data suggests that the prevalence of delirium seems to be higher in the subset of patients requiring NIV for acute respiratory failure (37%) than in a population of general medical inpatients (10–31%) [23]. The development of agitation and the deterioration of mental status, such as in delirious patients, decreases the ability to cooperate and tolerate NIV, potentially increasing the risks for NIV failure and subsequent intubation. The risk ratio of NIV failure in delirious patients was 2.12 as compared to that of nondelirious patients [23]. Elderly patients are particularly at risk of developing delirium and therefore routine screening for delirium would be beneficial, in addition to severity illness score. As poor prognosis in delirium patients, prevention of delirium was needed. Pain relief, early mobilization, improvement of sleep quality, and minimized noise were the promising methods to reduce delirium in NIV patients. Abdelgalel compared the effects of using dexmedetomidine and haloperidol for prevention of delirium during NIV in 90 adult intensive care patients of ASA physical status III and IV on NIV randomly allocated to three equal groups (Group D (30 patients) received dexmedetomidine, group H (30 patients) received haloperidol, and group P (30 patients) received normal saline infusion) [24]. Dexmedetomidine was more effective than haloperidol for prevention of delirium during NIV with lower incidence of endotracheal intubation and shorter ICU and hospital stay [24].

Sleep disruption was identified as a factor in late NIV failure. In mechanically ventilated patients, ventilator asynchrony may adversely affect sleep and there is evidence that in NIV patients, sleep is associated with more asynchrony and blood-oxygen desaturations than the awake state [25]. Environmental factors, mechanical ventilation, critical illness itself, and medication play an important role in sleep disruption in critically ill patients. Multiple studies indicated that impaired secretion of melatonin was observed in critically ill patients, which may be associated with the development of sleep deprivation and delirium. The administration and the sudden discontinuation of many medications can influence the wake–sleep-regulatory system by a direct effect on neurotransmitter and hormone activity. Benzodiazepines and opioids can reduce both SWS and REM sleep via GABA type A and opioid receptor stimulation, respectively. Additionally, opioids can cause delirium by decreasing acetylcholine and increasing dopamine and glutamate activity. Propofol suppresses the REM sleep stage and further worsens the poor sleep quality of these patients and might be associated with short-term (delirium) and long-term (post-traumatic stress disorder, PTSD) effects in critically ill patients.

Although the use of analgosedation in patients intolerant to NIV may have a strong rationale, the real benefit in the clinical practice is uncertain until the lack of large randomized controlled trials will endure. Sedation could be used in specific clinical setting only after a first non-pharmacological approach has been carried out to improve the patient's interaction/adaptation to ventilation.

Furthermore, the use of analgosedation cannot ignore the consideration of other aspects such as the level of experience of the medical and nursing staff, the use of clinical systems for determining/monitoring the level of pain, distress, and depth of sedation, as well as adequate pharmacovigilance. No single sedative agent is available that fulfills the criteria for an ideal drug and further studies are required to determine it. However, dexmedetomidine is noted as an emerging drug as a sedative in such patients. All patients receiving sedation should be monitored and evaluated at a frequent interval and dose needs to be titrated as required.

Further study, especially randomized controlled trial or active control trial, will be required in the future.

References

1. Carlucci A, Richard J-C, Wysocki M, Lepage E, Brochard L. Noninvasive versus conventional mechanical ventilation an epidemiologic survey and the SRLF collaborative group on mechanical ventilation. Am J Respir Crit Care Med. 2001;163(4):874–80.
2. Pisani L, Bianco GL, Pugliesi M, Tramarin J, Gregoretti C. Sedation and analgesia during noninvasive ventilation (NIV). In: Practical trends in anesthesia and intensive care 2017. Springer; 2017. https://doi.org/10.1007/978-3-319-61325-3_9.
3. Nava S, Hill N. Non-invasive ventilation in acute respiratory failure. Lancet. 2009;374(9685):250–9. https://doi.org/10.1016/S0140-6736(09)60496-7.
4. Muriel A, et al. Impact of sedation and analgesia during noninvasive positive pressure ventilation on outcome: a marginal structural model causal analysis. Intensive Care Med. 2015;41:1586–600. https://doi.org/10.1007/s00134-015-3854-6.
5. Devlin JW, Nava S, Fong JJ, Bahhady I, Hill NS. Survey of sedation practices during noninvasive positive-pressure ventilation to treat acute respiratory failure. Crit Care Med. 2007;35(10):2298–302. https://doi.org/10.1097/01.CCM.0000284512.21942.F8.
6. Conti G, Hill NS, Nava S. Is sedation safe and beneficial in patients receiving NIV? No. Intensive Care Med. 2015;41:1692–5. https://doi.org/10.1007/s00134-015-3915-x.
7. Longrois D, et al. Sedation in non-invasive ventilation: do we know what to do (and why)? Multidiscip Respir Med. 2014;9:56. https://doi.org/10.1186/2049-6958-9-56.
8. Devlin JW, et al. Clinical practice guidelines for the prevention and Management of Pain, agitation/sedation, delirium, immobility, and sleep disruption in adult patients in the ICU. Crit Care Med. 2018;46(9):e825–73. https://doi.org/10.1097/CCM.0000000000003299.
9. Marra A, Ely EW, Pandharipande PP, Patel MB. The ABCDEF bundle in critical care. Crit Care Clin. 2017;33:225–43.
10. Pandharipande P, et al. Lorazepam is an independent risk factor for transitioning to delirium in intensive care unit patients. Anesthesiology. 2006;104(1):21–6. https://doi.org/10.1097/00000542-200601000-00005.
11. Cavaliere F, et al. A low-dose remifentanil infusion is well tolerated for sedation in mechanically ventilated, critically-ill patients. Can J Anesth. 2002;49(10):1088–94. https://doi.org/10.1007/BF03017909.
12. Conti G, et al. Sedation with sufentanil in patients receiving pressure support ventilation has no effects on respiration: a pilot study. Can J Anesth. 2004;51(5):494–9. https://doi.org/10.1007/BF03018315.
13. Costa R, et al. Remifentanil effects on respiratory drive and timing during pressure support ventilation and neurally adjusted ventilatory assist. Respir Physiol Neurobiol. 2017;244:10–6. https://doi.org/10.1016/j.resp.2017.06.007.
14. Vaschetto R, et al. Effects of propofol on patient-ventilator synchrony and interaction during pressure support ventilation and neurally adjusted ventilatory assist. Crit Care Med. 2014;42(1):74–82. https://doi.org/10.1097/CCM.0b013e31829e53dc.
15. Clouzeau B, et al. Target-controlled infusion of propofol for sedation in patients with non-invasive ventilation failure due to low tolerance: a preliminary study. Intensive Care Med. 2010;36:1675–80. https://doi.org/10.1007/s00134-010-1904-7.
16. Senoglu N, et al. Sedation during noninvasive mechanical ventilation with dexmedetomidine or midazolam: a randomized, double-blind, prospective study. Curr Ther Res Clin Exp. 2010;76:3. https://doi.org/10.1016/j.curtheres.2010.06.003.
17. Huang Z, Chen Y s, Yang Z l, Liu J y. Dexmedetomidine versus midazolam for the sedation of patients with non-invasive ventilation failure. Intern Med. 2012;51(17):2299–305. https://doi.org/10.2169/internalmedicine.51.7810.
18. Devlin JW, et al. Efficacy and safety of early dexmedetomidine during noninvasive ventilation for patients with acute respiratory failure: a randomized, double-blind, placebo-controlled pilot study. Chest. 2014;145(6):1204–12. https://doi.org/10.1378/chest.13-1448.
19. Shutes BL, Gee SW, Sargel CL, Fink KA, Tobias JD. Dexmedetomidine as single continuous sedative during noninvasive ventilation: typical usage, hemodynamic effects, and withdrawal. Pediatr Crit Care Med. 2018;19(4):287–97. https://doi.org/10.1097/PCC.0000000000001451.
20. Venkatraman R, Hungerford JL, Hall MW, Moore-Clingenpeel M, Tobias JD. Dexmedetomidine for sedation during noninvasive ventilation in Pediatric patients*. Pediatr Crit Care Med. 2017;18(9):831–7. https://doi.org/10.1097/PCC.0000000000001226.
21. Piastra M, et al. Dexmedetomidine is effective and safe during NIV in infants and young children with acute respiratory failure. BMC Pediatr. 2018;18:282. https://doi.org/10.1186/s12887-018-1256-y.
22. Ni YN, Wang T, Yu H, Liang BM, Liang ZA. The effect of sedation and/or analgesia as rescue treat-

ment during noninvasive positive pressure ventilation in the patients with Interface intolerance after Extubation. BMC Pulm Med. 2017;17:125. https://doi.org/10.1186/s12890-017-0469-4.

23. Charlesworth M, Elliott MW, Holmes JD. Noninvasive positive pressure ventilation for acute respiratory failure in delirious patients: understudied, underreported, or underappreciated? A systematic review and meta-analysis. Lung. 2012;190:597–603. https://doi.org/10.1007/s00408-012-9403-y.

24. Abdelgalel EF. Dexmedetomidine versus haloperidol for prevention of delirium during non-invasive mechanical ventilation. Egypt J Anaesth. 2016;32:4, 473–81. https://doi.org/10.1016/j.egja.2016.05.008.

25. Fanfulla F, et al. Effect of sleep on patient/ventilator asynchrony in patients undergoing chronic non-invasive mechanical ventilation. Respir Med. 2007;101(8):1702–7.   https://doi.org/10.1016/j.rmed.2007.02.026.

Part VII

Non-invasive Mechanical Ventilation in Do Not Endotracheal Intubation Order and Palliative Care

Palliative Use of Non-invasive Ventilation

Giuseppe Servillo and Pasquale Buonanno

Contents

20.1 Introduction

Non-invasive ventilation (NIV) has been widely investigated in respiratory failure and its beneficial effects have been demonstrated in both hypercapnic and hypoxemic conditions; furthermore, NIV has assumed an important role to support patient's breathing after extubation [1]. Only few studies have been so far performed to evaluate its role in the palliative care setting which is extremely complex; in fact, end-of-life cannot be defined only by clinical parameters because ethical and psychological elements intertwine, making every medical decision more difficult. Furthermore, not only the patient's needs have to be taken into account, but also the relatives' perspective has to be considered. Death, in fact, just like birth, is far from being a personal event: it is a fundamental moment of family life [2].

It is very important to consider if NIV can actually improve quality of life in terminal patients or it just prolongs life without beneficial effects on patients' perception of symptoms [3].

The palliative use of NIV has so far investigated mainly in patients affected by solid or hematological cancers and patients suffering from end-stage chronic respiratory diseases [4].

In the clinical setting of a progressive condition with a poor prognosis, it is important to plan in advance with the patient and his relatives the interventions to carry out in the final stages of the disease in order to make every decision really informed and conscious.

There are different ways to handle with end-of-life and they should be chosen not only according to the patient wishes but also on the basis of local legislation:

- Withdrawal: the discontinuation of treatments in course in order not to prolong life anymore.
- Withholding: life-sustaining therapies (e.g., vasoactive drugs, continuous renal replace-

G. Servillo · P. Buonanno (✉)
Department of Neurosciences and Reproductive and Odontostomatological Sciences, University of Naples "Federico II", Naples, Italy

ment therapy, intubation) are not in course and they are decided not to be started.

- Euthanasia: an active and deliberate delivery of lethal substances by a physician when patient expresses the will to put an end to his intolerable symptoms.
- Physician-assisted suicide: the physician facilitates patient's death giving him all the necessary means and/or information (e.g., prescribing drugs and giving information about the lethal dose, route of administration, etc.).

End-of-life decisions are often influenced by many factors: one of the most important elements is the religion belief of the patient and the religion belief of the health care provider too. The skills and the experience of the physician are also very important in order to be able to manage a variety of situations which need tailored treatment according to the symptoms and wishes of the patients and relatives. Furthermore, national laws and guidelines are considerably different among the states and so the conclusions drawn by all the studies could not be generally applicable [5, 6].

In the final stage of diseases like end-stage chronic obstructive pulmonary disease (COPD), pulmonary fibrosis, amyotrophic lateral sclerosis, and cancer, many factors can influence the decisions about the treatment to choose: short life expectancy, a poor prognosis, and a low probability to get through the acute exacerbation of the disease [7].

NIV could have a beneficial application mainly in three groups of terminal patients: patients who want to undergo all available life-supporting treatments; patients who set limits to the possible interventions (e.g., do not intubate (DNI) order), and patients who want to receive comfort measures only (CMO).

20.2　End-Stage Chronic Respiratory Disease

An advanced care planning is fundamental in all end-of-life settings and the basic premise is a correct information of the patients and his family about the evolution and the prognosis of the disease; it is dramatically important to explain all the possible treatments and also the available palliative interventions to manage the symptoms and their effectiveness. It has been demonstrated that COPD patients who used informative material as audiocassette and booklet explaining the technique, advantages, and risks of mechanical ventilation have been effectively helped to make a decision [8].

Many studies underlined that communication is widely overlooked and the decision about the management of the latest phases of the life are delayed in a moment when the patient has not the possibility to express his wishes so medical staff generally takes decisions for him [7, 9, 10].

Some studies demonstrated that the compliance of patients is strictly dependent on the results the treatments are expected to produce; in fact, if COPD patients and those affected by cancer or cardiogenic pulmonary edema see the chance to restore their previous status, they are more likely to accept low-burden treatments but not highly invasive procedures. Furthermore, if the treatment cannot lead the patient back to his previous condition but could determine a significant reduction of functional or cognitive status, it is often refused even if it is not highly invasive [11].

NIV should be considered for both patients setting boundaries to the treatments, as it represents a low invasive life support who can help patients refusing intubation, and for CMO patients who want to have some relief from dyspnea [3]. The use and the trust in NIV to improve respiratory symptoms are different among the physicians on the basis of their background: intensive care physicians are generally less confident in the effectiveness of NIV in the end-of-life setting compared to pulmonologists. The reason could be that intensive care professionals are focused on the acute episode and they do not take into account the previous condition of the patients while pulmonologists follow the patients during the evolution and the progression of the disease and they can really appreciate the improvement of patients' condition after the NIV treatment with more realistic expectations [12].

The use of NIV ventilation is still debated mainly in CMO patients: in fact, NIV is a type of mechanical ventilation and it is difficult to establish if it can unnecessarily prolong life or simply alleviate dyspnea. This is an important issue both for physician, who could deny NIV in these situations as it is a mechanical support, and for patients, who could be afraid to prolong their suffering. The importance of a correct communication is crucial as the patient should be informed of the difference between NIV and intubation and their impact on life expectancy and symptoms relief. The expression "do not noninvasively ventilate order" could be added to DNI order to underline the patient's wish not to undergo NIV too.

More studies are needed especially to determine the target of NIV in the end-of-life scenario so patients and relatives could be clear which are the beneficial effects they have to expect in order to avoid an undesired prolongation of life and physical and psychological stress [13, 14]. The primary aims of NIV in the end-of-life are the control of symptoms (i.e., dyspnea) and sometimes to give patient an additional time to talk with his beloved persons and to settle his affairs [15].

The Task Force on the "Palliation Use of NIV" from the Society of Critical Care Medicine set the targets that NIV has to achieve according to the different patients and the invasiveness of treatments they accept to receive. The primary aim of NIV in CMO patients is to relieve dyspnea so if any form of discomfort raises during NIV treatment, it should be discontinued and other means of CMO have to be initiated. As the primary aim in CMO patients is to reduce symptoms to improve patient's comfort in the last phases of his life, NIV should not be started in unconscious patients who would not be aware of its positive effects [16, 17]. NIV can be used to allow patient's transfer to his own home where he can die surrounded by his family: also, this could be considered a palliative use of NIV.

NIV has to be evaluated regularly not only to determine the effectiveness of the treatment but also because patient could change his mind about the level of support he wants to receive, thus passing from a category to another.

A European survey underlined that the use of NIV is primarily reserved to DNI patients but it is rarely proposed to CMO patients because it is a mechanical support and consequently considered too invasive for these kind of patients [7].

The choice of NIV in patients who set limits to the treatments they want to undergo and in CMO patients is very difficult as no RCTs have so far conducted in this type of patients which are usually excluded from trials; very few specific studies have been so far performed about the palliative use of NIV and this make physicians' choice to start NIV in these conditions very difficult and the potential benefits has to be inferred by other studies conducted not in the end-of-life setting which demonstrated the effectiveness of NIV in reducing dyspnea in acute respiratory failure in COPD and solid cancer patients [18, 19]. Patient's information about NIV has to include not only the potential benefits but also the possible risks such as pneumothorax, eye irritation, hemodynamic instability, gastrointestinal distension, and patient–ventilator asynchronies [20].

COPD is the most common chronic respiratory pathology and, consequently, the palliative use of NIV in this condition has been more deeply studied; in fact, COPD exacerbations are commonly treated with NIV and it represents the fundamental therapeutic choice in these situations [3]. The use of NIV in other chronic respiratory diseases such as neuromuscular and neurological pathologies is debated because they are degenerative conditions with no hope of improvement; in these cases, the ethical issue is thornier because in the early stages, NIV can prolong life but in the last phases, patients became totally dependent on the respiratory support. Patients generally choose to keep on using NIV even if tracheostomy represents the best option in this type of patient not only to ensure the respiratory support but also to better manage the secretions and by consequence to prevent airway infections [21–23]. One of the chronic respiratory conditions in which NIV has been poorly investigated is pulmonary fibrosis; acute respiratory failure is a common event in the natural history of the disease and the use of NIV, even if it could bring advantages compared to oxygen and medical therapy, is far from being elucidated [24, 25].

20.3　Neoplastic Disease

The development of both pharmacological and radiological therapies has dramatically changed the prognosis of oncological patients; furthermore, hematopoietic stem cells and bone marrow transplantation have represented a cornerstone in the treatment of hematological malignancies. Even if these treatments can effectively influence the course of the disease, they have important adverse effects such as immunosuppression and drug-related toxicity which can impair organ function, thus making these patients more fragile. Cancer patients can undergo respiratory failure which represents one of the most important causes of intensive care unit admission in the oncological population [26–28]. The admission of cancer patients in ICU is a matter of debate because the chance to get through the acute episode should be carefully evaluated; in fact, the mortality of invasively ventilated patients is still high ~75–80% and the overall reduction of mortality for the other oncological patients in ICU has many explanation: a better choice about admission criteria in ICU, early admission for patients more prone to take advantage from intensive cares, and a better knowledge of the pathophysiology and complications of this type of patients [27, 29–31]. The high mortality of patients undergone mechanical ventilation questions if it is appropriate to admit in ICU such patients and raises the issue to alleviate end-of-life symptoms as respiratory fatigue.

NIV has demonstrated to effectively reduce ICU mortality and improve gas exchange during the episodes of respiratory failure; it can reduce the need of tracheal intubation and it is a huge advantage for cancer patients. In fact, tracheal intubation is an invasive procedure which makes the patient more prone to develop airway infections such as ventilator-acquired pneumonia and this is particularly true for the oncological population which is generally immunosuppressed [32–34].

Many studies tried to evaluate the advantages and drawbacks of the different NIV devices; Helmet is one of the most tolerate interface with the lower risk of skin injury but it could lead to an excessive CO_2 rebreathing if not properly set and it should be harmful especially for hypercapnic patients [35, 36].

Cancer patients who decided not to be intubated are often denied the possibility of NIV because it is considered a mechanical respiratory support; thereby, many episodes of acute respiratory failure, which could be settled by NIV, are not treated. Furthermore, even in the end-of life scenario, NIV can help decrease the respiratory fatigue and reduce opioids dosage, thus having a fundamental palliative function [37].

The most appropriate setting for NIV in end-of-life depends on many factors; for example, if patient wishes to receive all the support and accepts to be intubated, ICU represents the best place to perform NIV as intubation could be promptly ensured. Even the severity of symptoms influences the setting as a more severe respiratory impairment and a more complex global condition need more trained health care professionals [38]. Hospices or respiratory units are probably the most suitable location to perform NIV in DNI and CMO patients because these are environments where patient can be surrounded by his relatives and friends till the end and he can receive the most appropriate treatment in the very last phases of his disease by specialized health care providers.

NIV is a promising palliative treatment for respiratory symptoms such as dyspnea in end-of-life patients but, if not properly used, it could become a dramatic source of discomfort, thus increasing physical and psychological suffering.

References

1. Rochwerg B, Brochard L, Elliott MW, Hess D, Hill NS, Nava S, Navalesi P Members Of The Steering Committee, Antonelli M, Brozek J, Conti G, Ferrer M, Guntupalli K, Jaber S, Keenan S, Mancebo J, Mehta S, Raoof S Members Of The Task Force.

Official ERS/ATS clinical practice guidelines: noninvasive ventilation for acute respiratory failure. Eur Respir J. 2017;50(2):1602426. https://doi.org/10.1183/13993003.02426-2016.

2. Akgün KM. Palliative and end-of-life care for patients with malignancy. Clin Chest Med. 2017;38(2):363–76. https://doi.org/10.1016/j.ccm.2016.12.010.

3. Curtis JR, Cook DJ, Sinuff T, et al. Noninvasive positive pressure ventilation in critical and palliative care settings: understanding the goals of therapy. Crit Care Med. 2007;35:932–9.

4. Nava S, Ferrer M, Esquinas A, Scala R, Groff P, Cosentini R, Guido D, Lin CH, Cuomo AM, Grassi M. Palliative use of non-invasive ventilation in end-of-life patients with solid tumours: a randomised feasibility trial. Lancet Oncol. 2013;14(3):219–27. https://doi.org/10.1016/S1470-2045(13)70009-3. Epub 2013 Feb 11

5. Nyman DJ, Eidelman LA, Sprung CL. Euthanasia. Crit Care Clin. 1996;12(1):85–96. https://doi.org/10.1016/s0749-0704(05)70216-5.

6. McClelland W, Goligher EC. Withholding or withdrawing life support versus physician-assisted death: a distinction with a difference? Curr Opin Anaesthesiol. 2019;32(2):184–9. https://doi.org/10.1097/ACO.0000000000000686.

7. Nava S, Sturani C, Hartl S, et al. End-of-life decision-making in respiratory intermediate care units: a European survey. Eur Respir J. 2007;30:156–64.

8. Dales RE, O'Connor A, Hebert P, Sullivan K, McKim D, Llewellyn-Thomas H. Intubation and mechanical ventilation for COPD: development of an instrument to elicit patient preferences. Chest. 1999;116:792–800.

9. Sprung CL, Cohen SL, Sjokvist P, et al. End-of-life practices in European intensive care units: the ethicus study. JAMA. 2003;290:790–7.

10. Abbott KH, Sago JG, Breen CM, Abernethy AP, Tulsky JA. Families looking back: one year after discussion of withdrawal or withholding of life-sustaining support. Crit Care Med. 2001;29:197–201.

11. Fried TR, Bradley EH, Towle VR, Allore H. Understanding the treatment preferences of seriously ill patients. N Engl J Med. 2002;346:1061–6.

12. Sinuff T, Cook DJ, Keenan SP, et al. Noninvasive ventilation for acute respiratory failure near the end of life. Crit Care Med. 2008;36:789–94.

13. Curtis S, Hill NS, Brennan J, Garpestad E, Nava S. Noninvasive ventilation in acute respiratory failure. Crit Care Med. 2007;35:2402–7.

14. Truog RD, Campbell ML, Curtis JR, et al. Recommendations for end-of-life care in the intensive care unit: a consensus statement by the American academy of critical care medicine. Crit Care Med. 2008;36:953–63.

15. Freichels T. Palliative ventilatory support: use of non-invasive pressure support ventilation in terminal respiratory insufficiency. Am J Crit Care. 1994;3:6–10.

16. International Consensus Conferences in Intensive Care Medicine. Noninvasive positive pressure ventilation in acute respiratory failure. Am J Respir Crit Care Med. 2001;163:283–91.

17. Scala R, Nava S, Conti G, et al. Noninvasive versus conventional ventilation to treat hypercapnic encephalopathy in chronic obstructive pulmonary disease. Intensive Care Med. 2007;33:2101–8.

18. Bott J, Carroll MP, Conway JH, et al. Randomized controlled trial of nasal ventilation in acute ventilatory failure due to chronic obstructive airways disease. Lancet. 1993;341:1555–7.

19. Cuomo A, Delmastro M, Ceriana P, et al. Noninvasive mechanical ventilation as a palliative treatment of acute respiratory failure in patients with end-stage solid cancer. Palliat Med. 2004;18:602–10.

20. Mehta S, Hill NS. Noninvasive ventilation. Am J Respir Crit Care Med. 2001;163:540–77.

21. Simonds AK. Ethics and decision making in end stage lung disease. Thorax. 2003;58:272–7.

22. Polkey MI, Lyall RA, Davidson AC, Leigh PN, Moxham J. Ethical and clinical issues in the use of home non-invasive mechanical ventilation for the palliation of breathlessness in motor neurone disease. Thorax. 1999;54:367–71.

23. Hess DR. Noninvasive ventilation in neuromuscular disease: equipment and application. Respir Care. 2006;51:896–911.

24. Stern JB, Mal H, Groussard O, et al. Prognosis of patients with advanced idiopathic pulmonary fibrosis requiring mechanical ventilation for acute respiratory failure. Chest. 2001;120:213–9.

25. Blivet S, Philit F, Sab JM, et al. Outcome of patients with idiopathic pulmonary fibrosis admitted to the ICU for respiratory failure. Chest. 2001;120:209–12.

26. Ewig S, Torres A, Riquelme R, et al. Pulmonary complications in patients with haematological malignancies treated at a respiratory ICU. Eur Respir J. 1988;12:116–22.

27. Kress JP, Christenson J, Pohlman AS, Linkin DR, Hall JB. Outcomes of critically ill cancer patients in a university hospital setting. Am J Respir Crit Care Med. 1999;160:1957–61.

28. Chaflin DB, Carlon GC. Age and utilization of ICU resources of critically ill cancer patients. Crit Care Med. 1990;18:694–8.

29. Kroschinsky F, Weise M, Illmer T, et al. Outcome and prognostic features of ICU treatment in patients with haematological malignancies. Intensive Care Med. 2002;28:1294–300.

30. Adam AK, Soubani AO. Outcome and prognostic factors of lung cancer patients admitted to the medical intensive care unit. Eur Respir J. 2008;31:47–53.

31. Schonfeld N, Timsit JF. Overcoming a stigma: the lung cancer patient in the intensive care unit. Eur Respir J. 2008;31:3–5.

32. Fagon JY, Chastre J, Domart Y, et al. Nosocomial pneumonia in patients receiving continuous mechanical ventilation. Prospective analysis of 52 episodes with use of protected specimen brush and quantitative culture techniques. Am Rev Respir Dis. 1989;139:877–84.

33. Elpern EH, Scott MG, Petro L, Ries MH. Pulmonary aspiration in mechanically ventilated patients with tracheostomies. Chest. 1994;105:563–6.
34. Hilbert G, Gruson D, Vargas F, et al. Noninvasive ventilation in immunodepressed patients with pulmonary infiltrates, fever and acute respiratory failure. N Engl J Med. 2001;344:481–7.
35. Hill NS. Noninvasive ventilation for immunocompromised patients. N Engl J Med. 2001;344:522–4.
36. Navalesi P, Costa R, Ceriana P, et al. Non-invasive ventilation in chronic obstructive pulmonary disease patients: helmet versus facial mask. Intensive Care Med. 2007;33:74–81.
37. Nava S, Esquinas A, Ferrer M, et al. Multicenter, randomised study of the use of non-invasive ventilation (NIV) vs oxygen therapy (O2) in reducing dyspnea in end-stage solid cancer patients with respiratory failure and distress. Eur Respir J. 2007;30(Suppl. 51):204s.
38. Carlucci A, Delmastro M, Rubini F, Fracchia C, Nava S. Changes in the practice of non-invasive ventilation in treating COPD patients over 8 years. Intensive Care Med. 2003;29:419–25.

Use of Non-invasive Mechanical Ventilation in Older Patients

21

Nicola Vargas, Loredana Tibullo, Angela Pagano, Erminia Ramponi, and Stefano Badolato

Contents

21.1 Introduction

Treatment with non-invasive ventilation (NIV) in older patients is different from the other adult patients, and if yes, why? This first question concerns some biological features linked to ageing, such as structural and functional lung changes and frailty. For some very frail older patients, intubation may be considered a questionable option. On the other hand, we know that the prognosis of severely frail older patients with respiratory failure may be strongly unfavourable if they were intubated. For these reasons, NIV in the last years has been considered a valid therapeutic alternative. But the second question is: is there yet a guideline specific for elderly patients? Do current guidelines refer to studies that include elderly patients with ageing over 80 years? The essential RTCs at the base of the guideline and recommendations of how to use NIV have been planned on 'binary option' (NIV or no NIV), and only some of these included patients with age much more than 75 years. In this chapter, the authors analyse all these aspects with a specific evaluation of older patients in the context of Do not intubate (DNI) and in the emergency room.

21.2 Structural and Functional Changes with Ageing

The respiratory system with ageing faces two kinds of changes related to structural such as thoracic cage, lung and muscles and those related to gas exchange. The increased stiffness due to osteoporosis, shortening of the thoracic vertebrae

N. Vargas (✉) · A. Pagano · E. Ramponi ·
S. Badolato
Medicine Ward and Emergency Department, San
Giuliano Hospital, Giugliano, Italy

L. Tibullo
Medicine Department, San Giuseppe Moscati
Hospital, Avellino, Italy

and kyphosis of the chest wall reduce the elastic load during inspiration and the ability to expand during inspiration. Ageing leads to the reduction of the vital capacity and an increase of residual volume. There is a heterogeneity of the ventilation-perfusion ratio and a reduction of the lung carbon monoxide (DCLO) with subsequent reduction in PAO_2 [1].

21.3 Frailty

Frailty is a clinical state characterised by a decrease of an individual's homeostatic reserves and is responsible for enhanced vulnerability to endogenous and exogenous stressors. Such extreme vulnerability conditions expose individuals to an increased risk of adverse health-related outcomes [2]. The incidence of frailty is very high in older patients. The prevalence of frailty increases with age, independently of the assessment instrument and ranges between 4% and 59% in community-dwelling elderly populations and is higher in women than in men [3]. Furthermore, the prevalence rate in a population depends on chronic diseases, including depression, nutritional status, and inherently socioeconomic background and education. Respiratory failure is a significant stressor, and its impact on the prognosis depends on the grade of frailty. We Know that frailty present before a critical illness may be worse and that the same critical conditions could increase the prevalence of the frailty [4]. In the last time, the prognosis of older patients hospitalised for COVID-19 nonsurvivors was more often frail, worse functional status, higher comorbidity burden, and delirium at admission [5]. The classic image of how elder patients have been classified accordingly with a grade of frailty has been provided by the Clinical Frailty Scale (CFS) as modified in 2007 (Fig. 21.1). Patients with scores from one to three

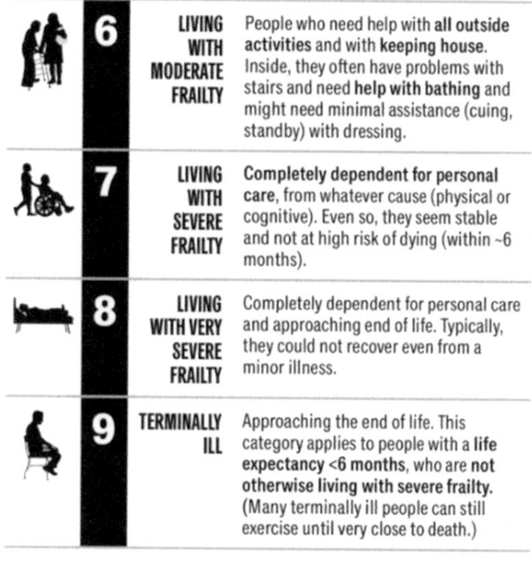

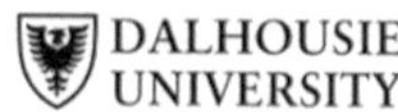

Fig. 21.1 Clinical frailty scale. 7 © 2007–2009. Version 1.2

are considered frail, four are pre-frail or vulnerable, and five to nine are considered frail. This tool is a way to summarise an older adult's overall level of fitness or frailty after being evaluated by an experienced clinician [6]. Generally, on this scale, the point from seven to nine is that ICU physicians examined to establish if the patients should not be intubated in case of critical illness and respiratory failure in the emergency room. Generally, frailty assessments are performed as comprehensive geriatric assessments. They require active patient participation, absent in most acutely admitted or critically ill patients. The CFS is considered a good instrument, and it can give a more holistic impression of the patient's condition before intensive care unit admission [7].

21.4 Very Old Patients and Do Not Intubate (DNI) Order

In 2011, their randomised controlled trial on NIV in hypercapnic respiratory failure in elderly patients with age >75 years showed positive results of the study on outcome on the mortality of the elder cohort considered. The authors concluded that the effects showed by their research highlighted the importance of using NIV not only as a palliative measure but also as preferential treatment when intubation is either not wanted by the patient or questionable for the physician [8]. However, Schortgen et al. [9] successively demonstrated that the prognosis of very old DNI patients treated with NIV was acceptable 6 months after discharge from the hospital. Physicians consider mechanical ventilation a questionable option in some daily (do not intubate) DNI-related clinical scenarios. For example, an oldest-old patient is bedridden, dependent on daily activity, multimorbidity, and acute respiratory failure [10]. The oldest-old have increased mortality when admitted to ICU. The setting out of ICU as a half-open geriatric ward may allow a good option for the oldest and their family members [11]. The provision of non-

invasive ventilation in a well-equipped hospital ward as a viable alternative to the ICU for selected patients was shown by a meta-analysis in 2018 [12], although the impact of non-invasive ventilation in patients with comfort-measures-only orders remain largely unanswered. Vilarca et al. tried to answer the impact of NIV as a comfort measure only [13]. They studied two groups of DNI in the emergency department (ED). The first group included DNI-order related to a decision to withhold therapy. The second group included those for whom any treatment, including NIV, was provided for symptom relief. They found that the survival rate was 49% among DNI-status patients for whom NIV was used as a treatment in ED. Furthermore, NIV did not provide significant relief of symptoms in more than half the patients who received it for that purpose. For very old patients are valid, the recommendations of the Society of Critical Care Medicine charged a Task Force to guide the use of NIV in palliative care settings [14]:

'type 1' patients in whom NIV is life support with no limitation of therapy, the authors identified distinct goals for patients in palliative settings;

'type 2' scenario in which a patient has decided to forego intubation but still wants to receive salvage NIV therapy to survive the hospitalisation; and

'type 3' patients seek symptom alleviation, mainly dyspnoea, and survival is not a goal for these patients.

Often the older patient has a limited capacity in decision-making capacity. Family members of older incompe741\tent patients are increasingly playing an essential role in the decision-making process relating to medical treatment. There are two main essential areas of surrogate's law in Europe: in the absence of the advance directives, the role of family members is automatically accepted as surrogates by law and a legal representative appointed by a court [15].

21.5 Conclusion

We should not consider older patients as a binary intervention option (NIV, no-NIV, or DNI). The physicians should consider some specific features such as frailty and the context of their family before deciding on NIV treatment.

References

1. Janssens JP, Pache JC, Nicod LP. Physiological changes in respiratory function associated with ageing. Eur Respir J. 1999;13(1):197–205. https://doi.org/10.1034/j.1399-3003.1999.13a36.x.
2. Cesari M, Calvani R, Marzetti E. Frailty in older persons. Clin Geriatr Med. 2017;33(3):293–303. https://doi.org/10.1016/j.cger.2017.02.002. Epub 2017
3. Rohrmann S. Epidemiology of frailty in older people. Adv Exp Med Biol. 2020;1216:21–7. https://doi.org/10.1007/978-3-030-33330-0_3.
4. Brummel NE, Girard TD, Pandharipande PP, et al. Prevalence and course of frailty in survivors of critical illness. Crit Care Med. 2020;48(10):1419–26. https://doi.org/10.1097/CCM.0000000000004444.
5. Mendes A, Serratrice C, Herrmann FR, Genton L, Périvier S, Scheffler M, Fassier T, Huber P, Jacques MC, Prendki V, Roux X, Di Silvestro K, Trombert V, Harbarth S, Gold G, Graf CE, Zekry D. Predictors of In-hospital mortality in older patients with COVID-19: the COVID age study. J Am Med Dir Assoc. 2020;21(11):1546–1554.e3. https://doi.org/10.1016/j.jamda.2020.09.014. Epub 2020 Sep 15
6. Rockwood K, Song X, MacKnight C, et al. A global clinical measure of fitness and frailty in older people. CMAJ. 2005;173(5):489–95. https://doi.org/10.1503/cmaj.050051.
7. Flaatten H, Guidet B, Andersen FH, et al. Reliability of the clinical frailty scale in very elderly ICU patients: a prospective European study. Ann Intensive Care. 2021;11(1):22. Published 2021 Feb 3. https://doi.org/10.1186/s13613-021-00815-7.
8. Nava S, Grassi M, Fanfulla F, Domenighetti G, Carlucci A, Perren A, Dell'Orso D, Vitacca M, Ceriana P, Karakurt Z, Clini E. Noninvasive ventilation in elderly patients with acute hypercapnic respiratory failure: a randomised controlled trial. Age Ageing. 2011;40(4):444–50.
9. Schortgen F, Follin A, Piccari L, et al. Results of noninvasive ventilation in very old patients. Ann Intensive Care. 2012;2:5. https://doi.org/10.1186/2110-5820-2-5.
10. Vargas N, Tibullo L, Landi E, et al. Caring for critically ill oldest-old patients: a clinical review. Aging Clin Exp Res. 2017;29:833–45. https://doi.org/10.1007/s40520-016-0638-y.
11. Vargas N, Vargas M, Galluccio V, Carifi S, Villani C, Trasente V, Landi CA, Cirocco A, Di Grezia F. Noninvasive ventilation for very old patients with limitations to respiratory care in the half-open geriatric ward: experience on a consecutive cohort of patients. Aging Clin Exp Res. 2014;26(6):615–23. https://doi.org/10.1007/s40520-014-0223-1. Epub 2014 Apr 30
12. Wilson ME, Majzoub AM, Dobler CC, Curtis JR, Nayfeh T, Thorsteinsdottir B, Barwise AK, Tilburt JC, Gajic O, Montori VM, Murad MH. Noninvasive ventilation in patients with do-not-intubate and comfort-measures-only orders: a systematic review and meta-analysis. Crit Care Med. 2018;46(8):1209–16. https://doi.org/10.1097/CCM.0000000000003082.
13. Vilaça M, Aragão I, Cardoso T, Dias C, Cabral-Campello G. The role of noninvasive ventilation in patients with "do not intubate" order in the emergency setting. PLoS One. 2016;11(2):e0149649. https://doi.org/10.1371/journal.pone.0149649.
14. Rochwerg B, Brochard L, Elliott MW, Hess D, Hill NS, Nava S, Navalesi P, Antonelli M, Brozek J, Conti G, Ferrer M, Guntupalli K, Jaber S, Keenan S, Mancebo J, Mehta S, Raoof S. Official ERS/ATS clinical practise guidelines: noninvasive ventilation for acute respiratory failure. Eur Respir J. 2017;50(2):1602426. https://doi.org/10.1183/13993003.02426-2016.
15. Tibullo L, Esquinas AM, Vargas M, Fabbo A, Micillo F, Parisi A, Vargas N. Who gets to decide for the older patient with a limited decision-making capacity: a review of surrogacy laws in the European Union. Eur Geriatr Med. 2018;9(6):759–69. https://doi.org/10.1007/s41999-018-0121-8. Epub 2018 Oct 29

Use of Non-invasive Ventilation at the End of Life

22

Giuseppe Servillo, Servillo Andrea, and Vargas Maria

Contents

22.1 Introduction

Non-invasive ventilation (NIV) has been well described as effective in different patient populations, for example, hypercapnic respiratory failure due to exacerbations of chronic obstructive pulmonary disease (COPD), [1] hypoxic respiratory failure in immunocompromised hosts, [2] or cardiogenic pulmonary edema in the absence of acute coronary ischemia, [3] to cite the most common indications. Conceptually, the use of non-invasive ventilation can be divided into the following three categories [4]:

1 NIV as a part of "full-code" treatment (life support without preset limits).
2 NIV in patients with do-not-intubate orders (life support with preset limits).
3 NIV as a comfort measure in patients at the end of life (NIV ensuring comfort while dying).

Each category has specific goals of care, response to failure, and main points to communicate with the patient and/or family. Categories 2 and 3 can be defined as palliative NIV [5].

The goals of NIV in patients in category 1 are to alleviate symptoms of respiratory distress, improve oxygenation and/or ventilation, avoid intubation, and reduce the risk of mortality. Endotracheal intubation is performed if

G. Servillo (✉) · V. Maria
Department of Neurosciences, Reproductive and Odontostomatological Sciences, University of Naples "Federico II", Naples, Italy
e-mail: servillo@unina.it

S. Andrea
Department of Ophthalmology, University Vita-Salute, IRCCS Ospedale San Raffaele, Milan, Italy

G. Servillo, M. Vargas (eds.), *Non-invasive Mechanical Ventilation in Critical Care, Anesthesiology and Palliative Care*, https://doi.org/10.1007/978-3-031-36510-2_22

necessary. Patients in category 2 are those who decline endotracheal intubation or patients in whom clinicians feel that intubation would not meet the goals of care. In this group, the use of NIV achieves the same goals as it does in category 1, except that endotracheal intubation is not an option in cases where NIV is ineffective. The only purpose of NIV in category 3 is symptom palliation and patient comfort.

22.2 Patients Suitable of NIV at the End of Life

NIV is used in three general circumstances in patients close to death, all of which are likely to be encountered by palliative specialists [1]:

1. Patients who desire full, life-prolonging interventions, regardless of prognosis. If the patient's respiratory status deteriorates, intubation and ventilation are initiated.
2. Patients who want life-prolonging therapy but with limitations (e.g., patients with a "Do Not Intubate" order but otherwise want all attempts at life prolongation). Ideally, NPPV is used only if the etiology for the respiratory failure is thought to be reversible and is stopped if it is not producing the desired response or the patient is not tolerating NPPV. In practice, this may not be the case.
3. Dying patients with respiratory failure or dyspnea for palliative purposes. This category includes dying patients who have decided to forego life-prolonging therapies and wish to focus on comfort measures. NPPV can be used with the intention to reduce the work of breathing, to ease dyspnea, and to help maintain wakefulness by reducing the amount of opioids a patient needs to be comfortable. NPPV can also be used to prolong life for a short period to meet a patient's goals while otherwise providing a comfortable death (e.g., to allow time for family to visit). Unlike #2, the goal is not to bridge a patient through a reversible illness, but to forestall death to meet a specific goal.

22.3 Medical Decision Making and Withdrawing of NIV

- Patients in categories #1 & 2, as with all patients nearing the end of life, need ongoing discussions about their realistic prognosis, goals, and options.
- For dying patients with distressing dyspnea and comfort-only goals of care, opioids are first-line agents. For patients who need sedating doses of opioids to be comfortable, and who articulate a strong preference to be as awake as possible, it is reasonable to offer NPPV if the patient is in an environment which can accommodate it and the risks are acceptable to the patient, including the possibility that the dying process will be prolonged. Reassure patients that you can alleviate their symptoms even if NPPV is unhelpful or intolerable.
- For dying patients who wish to forestall death briefly for a specific goal, it is reasonable to start a trial of NPPV. Before initiating NPPV, it is important to discuss withdrawal of NPPV after the above goal has been achieved, and to caution the patient/family that NPPV might not be able to forestall death long enough as hoped.

22.4 Planning the Process of Withdrawal

Once a decision has been made to withdraw NIV, planning for the process should begin. The following flowcharts show the processes that should be followed for complete withdrawal and weaned withdrawal. At this stage, it is important to determine which professionals will be responsible for each task. In practice, professionals may be responsible for more than one task. The following responsibilities should be allocated:

- Co-ordinating the planning and process of withdrawal of NIV.
- Leading discussions with the patient and family.

- Ensuring adequate medications are prescribed and available at the location.
- Administering medications.
- Turning off or reducing pressures of NIV.
- Removing the NIV mask and, if appropriate, replacing with an O_2 mask.
- Providing emotional support to family and friends.
- Performing personal care after death (last offices).
- Completing death certificate.

22.5   Symptoms of Respiratory Distress At the End of Life and Their Relief

Respiratory distress is one of the most common symptoms seen in patients approaching the end of life. It leads to restrictions in quality of life and increases anxiety and fear [5, 6].

Terminal dyspnea is a manifestation of an irreversible process, such as carcinomatous lymphangitis in malignant diseases or advanced degenerative neuromuscular disease (amyotrophic lateral sclerosis).

The vast majority of patients with terminal cancer experience symptoms of respiratory distress at some point during the last 6 weeks of life, and they commonly report significantly increased dyspnea during the last 2 weeks [7]. In patients with a noncancer terminal diagnosis, such as COPD or chronic heart failure (CHF), the severity of respiratory distress can be greater; however, the severity remains relatively stable until death.

The mechanism underlying the relief of respiratory distress through non-invasive ventilation remains the same in all clinical situations [8]. NIV reduces the work of breathing by increasing transpulmonary pressure and reducing inspiratory muscle workloads. Gas exchange is improved by increasing alveolar ventilation, functional residual capacity, opening collapsed alveoli, reducing shunts, and improving the ventilation/perfusion (V/Q) ratio. Altogether, these mecha-

nisms result in a lower respiratory rate, reduced CO_2 retention, and an overall improvement of symptoms of respiratory distress.

22.6   Ethical Issues

Decisions about stopping treatment at the end of life are emotionally distressing and some may involve ethical dilemmas. Some members of the healthcare team or the patient's friends or family may find it difficult to contemplate withdrawal of a life-sustaining treatment. A common concern is that this may be tantamount to assisted suicide. However, the withdrawal of a medical treatment is not equivalent to actively hastening a patient's death. The withdrawal of the treatment, whether at the request of a competent patient or following a consideration of best interests in a patient who lacks capacity, allows the underlying disease to take its natural course, which had been temporarily delayed by the NIV. These issues need to be explained to all involved prior to withdrawal. This can be a distressing time for those close to the patient and staff involved in their care. The need for bereavement support should be addressed at an early opportunity. Staff support mechanisms, including debriefing sessions, need to be considered.

References

1. Keenan SP, Sinuff T, Cook DJ, et al. Which patients with acute exacerbation of chronic obstructive pulmonary disease benefit from noninvasive positive-pressure ventilation? A systematic review of the literature. Ann Intern Med. 2003;138:861–70.
2. Hilbert G, Gruson D, Vargas F, et al. Noninvasive ventilation in immunosuppressed patients with pulmonary infiltrates, fever, and acute respiratory failure. N Engl J Med. 2001;344:481–7.
3. Vital FMR, Ladeira MT, Atallah AN. Non-invasive positive pressure ventilation (CPAP or bilevel NPPV) for cardiogenic pulmonary oedema. Cochrane Database Syst Rev. 2013;5:CD005351.
4. Curtis JR, Cook DJ, Sinuff T, et al. Noninvasive positive pressure ventilation in critical and palliative care settings: understanding the goals of therapy. Crit Care Med. 2007;35:932–9.

5. Azoulay E, Demoule A, Jaber S, et al. Palliative non-invasive ventilation in patients with acute respiratory failure. Intensive Care Med. 2011;37:1250–7.
6. Kamal AH, Maguire JM, Wheeler JL, et al. Dyspnea review for the palliative care professional: assessment, burdens, and etiologies. J Palliat Med. 2011;14:1167–72.
7. Shreves A, Pour T. Emergency management of dyspnea in dying patients. Emerg Med Pract. 2013;15:1–19.
8. Mehta S, Hill NS. Noninvasive ventilation. Am J Respir Crit Care Med. 2001;163:540–77.

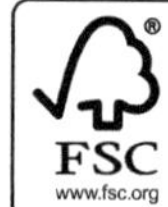